Warning: This book could be hazardous to your ideas of Western medicine and the American diet. It could severely disturb your comfortable, pasty lifestyle.

Any changes you make as a result of reading the opinions in this book constitute choices made by you, for which you are solely responsible.

If you need someone to blame for your life be sure to look in the mirror and don't read this book.

Health 101

Rated R

by

Nurse Rattschidt

Hykolonic Publications

Published in the United States and the United Kingdom by
Hykolonic Publications

ISBN 978-0-615-92230-0 (pbk.)
ISBN 978-1-4951-1850-0 (ebk.)

First edition 2014

Printed in the United States of America

Library of Congress Control Number: 2014940687

1 2 3 4 5 6 7 8 9 10

TABLE OF CONTENTS

PREFACE

Let me start off by saying that I try to ingest and acquire things that are as "natural" and as "organic" as possible. It is the chemical saturation in our environment (air, water, food...) that is the biggest offender of our ailments or sub-standard health.

Let me further say that a person must become informed and savvy, if not downright psychically knowledgeable about what absolutely takes on a healthy form for a person to ingest, breathe or wear. Marketing and the media do not give a rat's ass about your well-being. They care about their bank accounts.

The words "natural" and "organic" can legally be used on packaging and advertising. It is not a lie. You know why? Because everything is organic or natural. Rat shit is organic and natural. I don't intend to eat it or smear it on my face! (Of course, if they do prove rat shit is the miracle wrinkle cure I'll eat my words and be plastering those little pulverized rodent pebbles all over my body.) So I encourage people to always question advertising and packaging.

I'll give you an example….Decades ago when saturated fats, particularly butter, got a bad rep, there emerged the "natural, good for you vegetable oil" margarine. "Oh! Be heart smart! Eat a pound a day because it's good for you, it's vegetable oil!!" This product could legally state that it was indeed vegetable oil. On its own, in its natural "liquid at room temperature" state it is a good oil. But to put it in a cube so it can be spread on a piece of bleached white flour toast, it has to be solid. Yes? Yes. That means they take the vegetable oil molecule and add hydrogen atoms to it. Thus it becomes a hydrogenated oil….better known today as "trans-fats." A very bad dude now. It may not be the artery clogger that butter was made out to be, but instead it got linked to cancer. Isn't that better?

So in this book I will not be using euphemisms like natural and organic unless I damn well mean they are good for a person.

There is an R rating on this book, so viewer discretion is advised. There will be harsh language, hard truths, and scary scenarios. I'll throw some nudity in there if I can find a way.

Intro

It doesn't matter if I was born and raised in Leave It to Beaverland or in some atrociously dysfunctional, abusive trash pit. I will say that I have worked through many of the health/weight challenges that plague this society. I'm writing this book because there are things that I have found to be right and true and good, for me. If someone else can benefit from that knowledge then that would be a delightful side effect. My existence and my pocketbook do not depend on anyone purchasing or using this book. I enjoy it when people do the right things for themselves and I get vicarious pleasure out of their success. However, I have seen enough slothfulness and self abuse to have become completely jaded and cynical. If someone does not wish to help themselves then it is a waste of my time to try to help them.

That leads me to my second warning. If a person is not ready to grow some balls, grab the bull by the horns, resist all the brainwashed temptation and make some changes, then they should not read this book. It would be better for them to take that money and go buy some more Hydrogenated Puffy Cakes and Sodiumized Soda Drinks.

I would also like to add that I am not good at remembering names and dates and spewing out the exact resource of where I got my information. Nor do I want to. So don't take it on faith or a grain of salt or even as law. If you want resources, scientific research and studies, all that information is out there. Go after it. Get confirmation.....or prove me wrong. Either one is fine. I know what works for me and if you feel the need to find fault with that information then you obviously didn't take my advice not to read this book, or you may not be ready to get out of your comfort zone to make changes.

I will try to provide some reference material I find worthy, though. There are some good books out there that have been my bibles. I do hope you can benefit also. Just know this about the truth, especially when it comes to our health in this country.......it is not out in the open. It is typically locked away from public viewing. Always question the research you are reading. WHO WROTE THE REPORT? Then you'll find out what their agenda was when they did the study.

Chapter 1 — Oxygen: The Big Oh!!!

Remember the blonde joke? She had sticky notes all over that read "in" and "out". Someone asked what they were about and the other person said "Oh those are a reminder for her to keep breathing in and out". Well I'm here to tell you that that doesn't just apply to blondes. Trust me....I have sticky notes all over the damn place so I can remember to inhale and exhale. You would be surprised at how many people do not breathe correctly and sometimes not at all.

Oxygen is one of the most vital of all elements required by the body. You might say, "yeah, well Duh!" But for how simple, redundant and obvious a statement that may be it is surprising how overlooked that one component is. We take it for granted. I've watched people and even asked them if they hold their breath or breathe shallow. Quite often the answer is yes. I know this to apply to myself and even found it to be an inherited personality trait in my family. My statement above is not joking. I have to remind myself to breathe correctly.

Without oxygen, nutrients cannot be delivered to the cells. Let me give an example. A person with emphysema starts to lack the ability to exchange carbon dioxide out of the lungs for oxygen into the lungs, which then oxygenates the blood. This person could consume the most nutritious food sources on the planet but they would not be able to assimilate and utilize those precious life-giving nutrients without a delivery system. So it's like writing the most fabulous love letter (nutrients) and the postal system (oxygenated blood) is on strike. (Poor postal bastards are always getting a bad rep). That letter ain't gonna make it to the waiting lover.

So reminding ourselves to breathe in and out, regularly, is not so stupid after all. If a person checks themselves when they're stressed, or even just deep in thought, they might catch themselves holding their breath or breathing very shallow. Taking nice deep breaths that fill the belly and expand the lungs is required to get a good whopping dose of oxygen. It not only will nourish the cells, the side effect is it can relieve the effects of stress, some of which are chest pains which have sometimes been mistaken for angina (heart problems).

Your posture even goes a long way to assist the expansion of the lungs and more oxygen intake. Sitting up straight was not just something our parents bitched at us so they could hear themselves correcting us. It benefits the breathing thing as well as being beneficial to the spine (we'll cover the spine in a later chapter.) There was a study done of people who had suffered heart attacks. It was discovered that each of these people had poor rounded over posture that did not allow for maximum lung expansion, contributing to decreased oxygen intake and constricting (cheating) the heart. Gravity and stress start to get to us and we have to counter that pull downward by remembering to sit up straight and simply just breathing.

Another hidden oxygen robber is the "thief in the night"-----sleep apnea. I don't know why snoring and sleep apnea (stopping breathing) are so prevalent now, but it severely cheats oxygen to the brain. This leads to many ailments. Minimally, waking up tired, groggy, and irritable is one. Many people are prescribed mood stabilizers for mood swings when it could be as simple as getting a good night's sleep, which involves solving any snoring or apnea interruptions.

When the brain cannot get enough oxygen and the cycle of sleep is interrupted by bouts of gasping for air, it cannot enter into deep sleep and the dream states. Without the oxygen and the deep sleep it cannot successfully repair itself each night. This inability to repair itself has been linked to debilitating things such as diabetes, obesity, and Alzheimers just to name a few.

Our environment is already in an oxygen deficit what with all the pollution and destruction of plant life (which provides O2 to the air). Back in prehistoric times the oxygen level was much greater than now. To further scare the shit out of everyone (we will cover that in the shit list) cancer loves a low oxygen environment. So we not only have to worry about our own mechanism for utilizing oxygen (our lungs), we now get to worry about where to get enough of it.

A Note On Smoking:

Yeah, yeah, we've heard it all. I'm a non-smoker and even I get sick of hearing people telling me what to do and what's bad for me. No one wants to be told what to do. OK that's a given. But let me just say this. If you chose to keep smoking that is your right. No one is holding a gun to your head, so no one is to blame if the unspeakable happens, OK? It's not the tobacco company's fault. (Hey we don't sue the auto industry for the thousands of people who get killed in cars every day.) But here's what I've heard from smokers who have a defensive attitude about smoking. "Hey I love to smoke. I have no intentions of ever quitting. We all have to die so why not be happy until I do." Really? So you think that smoking is just a happy proposition and you just one day drop dead instantly with a smile on your face? Well let me tell you what I've seen. People who contract Chronic Obstructive Pulmonary Disease (COPD), Congestive Heart Failure (CHF), Emphysema and Lung Cancer (all diseases most likely to occur with smoking) can linger for years, even decades at great expense to insurance companies, Medi-Cal, Medicare, they end up living in nursing care homes, struggling every minute to breathe. Hooked up to oxygen machines and gasping because the mechanism in their lungs can't make the exchange anymore. It's long and drawn out. It's painful to watch them breathe. Every breathe is a fight. Even the end is not easy. It's horrible to watch. So I just wanted to clear up the misperception of "dying happy." Not likely.

In Conclusion:

1. If you have to put "in" and "out" sticky notes on your computer, your mirror or your forehead----Do It!

2. If you have to go to an ENT Doc (Ear, Nose & Throat) or get a sleep study to see what you do (or don't do) during the night----Do It!

3. If you have to strap a rod to your back to keep you upright----Do It!

4. If you have to quit smoking to protect your lungs----well that's up to you. You're a big kid. I don't have to preach the dangers of cigarette smoke, however I also know how hard it is to break habits.

5. If you have to trade that Snickers bar for a piece of celery to introduce higher oxygen content food into your body----then Do It!!!!

Chapter 2 — Water: Well, Well, Well, What a Deep Subject

Simple concept---Water. But I love it when people brush me off with "Oh I get plenty of fluids----I drink tea, juice, coffee, soda all day long." DOESN'T COUNT. The kidneys (hence the tissues) need pure H2O to flush them. That means nothing dissolved or dissipated in it. It will no longer have the regular osmotic factor to it. The kidneys are considered one of the master organs. Many imbalances can be traced to the kidneys as the core problem of things that can look like other organs and systems are compromised. Treat them good and many other functions can fall into place and even correct themselves.

In the old days edema (swelling) was treated by restricting water intake. WRONG! Being chincy with the water makes the kidneys go into DefCon 5 alert that the body is losing vital fluids. (It can only read the little stream of fluid passing through them, not the Lake Erie that has holed up in the cells.) So if minimal water is passing through the kidneys it sends an APB to the brain (pituitary) to send out an Anti-Diruetic Hormone (ADH) to stop any more loss of fluid. So it conserves even more fluid by sending it to the tissues, causing even more edema. This is what a normal kidney will do. Any damaged kidney is high medical risk factor and needs professional care.

Water also offers more oxygen. (Remember the big O?) A study was done with people trying to scale Mt. Everest. The higher the altitude the less the oxygen. People could not breathe at those high elevations and tried many oxygen replacing devices to no avail. It was discovered that if they increased their water intake they could breathe and climb higher. Yee-ha.

Let's look at juice. A "natural" fluid. Yes it's from fruit, a very good food source. But it is the sugars from several pieces of fruit compressed into a single serving. It's still sugar. Most diabetics know it's a no-no to overdo juices. I bet many a blood sugar reading has spiked because juice was consumed. It's better to just eat the piece of fruit.

Sodas. Here's where I know I'm going to get the most flack and resistance. Not only are sugars added, but sodiums (salt in many forms) and carbon dioxide compressed into one can. We're talking about a gas the kidneys really don't like and have to work overtime to break down, releasing bad by-products. That, plus the sodium does the opposite of hydrating the body. Sodas were not originally designed to be consumed all day long as a hydrating fluid source. They were supposed to be a treat. Now we act as if they are one of the basic four food groups and without them we would perish.

It could be argued that sodas have the essential sodium that is lost by the body during exertion, sweating and severe heat. Yes, the body does lose essential electrolytes like sodium and potassium during hard work and extreme sports activity. That's why the power drinks like Gatorade have become so popular. But my observation is that people who are consuming massive quantities of sodas are not expending extended periods of energy and sweat. If they are sweating it's because their bodies are insulated with about a hundred pounds of excess fat and walking from the car to the store to buy their 6-pack of soda was an extreme effort. But also remember this: Anything can be overdone. The argument to replace lost electrolytes is a good argument, however, even electrolytes can be in excess in the body. So too much consumption of electrolytes is not a good thing. There has to be an equal amount of water to dilute the electrolytes in the proper balance needed by the body.

If that isn't enough to screw with your mind, add this tidbit. Even water can be consumed to excess. Too much water will wash out all the electrolytes. The body is basically electrical. It needs the electrolytes to make the chemical conductions for the organs and systems to work like a well-oiled machine. Without those electrolytes this system will seize like that engine and shutdown.

If the electrolytes get completely washed out of the body it will first feel "high", sort of drunk and light-headed. Usually the next step would be seizures. The next occurrence could be coma. If this condition persists, then the next step is death.

The next argument regarding sugar content could be, "I choose sugar-free drinks." Yeah? Really? Do you really know what those sugar substitutes are made of? Do you want to know? Do you know what happens when those chemical compounds hit your internal 98.6 environment? It turns into a toxic substance. I've heard it compared to wood alcohol. Personally I'd opt for the regular sugar if I had no other choice but to choose between these two.

Now there's the subject of the caffeine in sodas, teas and coffee, especially if you like the high octane, fully leaded varieties. If you are prone to headaches, anxiety, insomnia and even mania, I have one word for you---HELLO!!!! Caffeine aggravates every one of those symptoms. Caffeine is also found in our beloved chocolate. Hey, I live in a glass house on this one folks. I am a coffee addict. But I can only handle so much caffeine before I bat a thousand on that checklist of side effects above, including the mania (due to popular opinion).

Another clue that a person is water deficient is if they are getting chronic headaches. This is a sign of dehydration. Sometimes relief from the headache wasn't from the aspirin or the ibuprofen but from the glass of water used to wash it down. In Chinese medicine a frontal headache is a message from the kidneys that they need water. (Got the T-shirt on this one too.) Before my alternative studies

I had developed chronic headaches. I then learned about the kidneys and water. Once I started drinking water the headaches disappeared. And since I'm such a terrible water drinker, I have to treat myself like a disobedient child. First thing in the morning I am not allowed to have my beloved breakfast until I consume 3 large glasses of water. I am hydrated for the day plus I get all that inconvenient peeing out of the way early on.

Now the dilemma is if you really want to treat those parched overworked kidneys to a good water quenching-----where do you acquire this miracle liquid? Our city waters are treated with chlorine and other chemicals. Bottled water has two downfalls: 1) It's not regulated so it very well could be tap water. 2) When liquid sits in plastic containers and is exposed
to heat, it releases an estrogen-like molecule. (That's an entire subject in itself.) So how do you know what's in that bottle?

Your best bet is if you have a well and have tested it for bacteria and other harmful substances. If you don't have a well then don't despair. I do believe that many filtering systems are a good choice and some are reasonably priced. I myself double filter my water. Yes I still worry.

Some caution on distilled water. I see many recommendations for use of drinking distilled water. It may be good for flushing impurities out of the body but it should only be used short term. Since distilled water has no minerals in it, it can pull the minerals out of a person's body. Long term this could cause deficiencies.

In conclusion:

1. Review your water intake. The recommended amount is 6 to 8 glasses a day. If you drink zero then be realistic. Can you get 3 or 4 in? That's a good start.

2. If you already are a water drinker, are you drinking too much? Too much could be washing out valuable electrolytes.

3. Are you a hard-core soda drinker? If you can't cut back, at least drink one whole glass of water for every can of soda consumed. That will still help minimize the load on the kidneys.

4. Do your best to find good clean water sources. More expensive is not a guarantee.

Chapter 3 — Nutrition: See if You Can Swallow This

The most basic analogy I have found is that the body is like a vehicle. It cannot run anywhere without fuel in it. So you have to put fuel into the vehicle, that's a given. Food is the body's fuel. So the question remains, are you going to put high octane into your tank or are you using Horrible Henry's gas? I guess it depends on whether you see yourself as a Maserati or some piece of shit Clunker.

The hard fact is that we all have to eat and it has to be quality IF you want an optimum running machine. You really are what you eat. (Is that why they keep calling me a prick down at the office?) There's also a good computer analogy here---garbage in, garbage out. So how can I accomplish this monumental task with the least amount of effort and discipline? I'm basically lazy. I cannot prescribe to fanaticism (that is unless sex is involved). So let's break it down into smaller components.

BALANCED DIET

We've all heard the balanced diet schpiel forever---yah, yah, blah, blah, blah. But there is validity to it. Basically you need proteins, whole grains, fruits and vegetables.

The trick is to get each one of these groups to be as close to its original form as possible. If you can eat a potato instead of Chef Blimpo's packaged potatoes au gratin in a box, good. If you can eat a fresh tomato (especially in a salad) instead of Porky's cream of tomato soup, good. Brown rice instead of pasta. An apple instead of fruit cocktail in a can. If you can begin to think like this and actually do it you are doing much better than the average American schmoe eating his Heart Attack on a Bun or Kidney Failure in a Box with a megasize side of fries with catsup (which is basically sugarized tomatoes).

Beef: Beef is easy. Although the reason it got a bad rep is because it wasn't raised properly. I will illustrate this more in the blood type section, but for now just know that corn is not the natural food for cows. When any creature consumes what is not their natural food their bodies produce toxins. These toxins then need to be corralled (excuse the pun). Their bodies produce fat to harbor those toxins. Hence the marbling in the meat. That's why THAT fat is not good for us. Otherwise meat is a terrific source of protein, B vitamins, iron and omega 3's. Animal flesh is also the only source of the 8 essential amino acids that our bodies cannot produce and need.

The other concern is the antibiotics and growth hormones given to our cattle. Anything our livestock consumes, we consume. The medical profession has already over prescribed antibiotics to our human population. We are getting a double dose if the animal has been given antibiotics also.

Note: Omega 3's are one of the most heart healthy, brain healthy, beneficial oils you can take. Omega 3's deserve their own chapter.

Fish: The only question here is, is it mercury free? Otherwise fish is a great source of protein and omega 3's.

Chicken and Turkey: Again, are they safe from hormones and antibiotics? If so they are wonderful sources of protein and other nutrients, such as Tryptophan which is the ingredient in hot milk that helps you fall asleep. (why do you think babies sleep right after they eat. Sleep helps their brains to grow so nature put a sedative in the main food source.)

Eggs: Another wonderful food that got a bad rep. First by the cholesterol found in the yolk and then the Salmonella scare. I never believed either one, personally. To this day I'd suck down a raw egg if I had no other food to eat. Hell I'll eat an egg any way, shape or form. I later heard that they found there were characteristics in the white of the egg that counteracted any effects of the cholesterol in the yoke. Did they make that national hoopla and say "Oops, we made a mistake"? Hell no. In other countries they have signs on their eggs in the store that announce "this is a heart smart food". Besides, cholesterol is a food source and is not necessarily bad. We are the only country that makes eggs a bad guy. And that Salmonella thing? What were they doing, feeding the chickens shit soup? How the fuck does Salmonella get into an enclosed egg in the first place!?

Note: If you have high cholesterol I suggest you do a food diary and really look at what you are consuming. It's critical to be brutally honest. If you find you are eating fast foods or canned and packaged foods (processed), there are additives that are not good nutritious food sources. Read the labels. Do you know what half of those ingredients are? Hell I don't. What I do know is there is hydrogenated fats (remember those from the introduction?) added along with different kinds of starches and sugars you don't need. Are you eating things that contain bleached four, such as crackers, cookies, breads, cereals, bagels and pasta to name a few? Do you choose margarine instead of butter? Margarine IS hydrogenated oil. What is your intake of sugar? Count every soda, sweetened ice tea and Gatorade along with the obvious sweets like pastries, ice cream and yogurt. (Yes yogurt can be loaded with sugar). Do you eat fried foods? Do you have a stressful lifestyle? Do you get a solid night's sleep or is it interrupted by frequent waking, snoring or sleep apnea? Are you overweight? If you answer yes to these questions then it is more likely these factors have contributed to an elevated cholesterol level rather than a few eggs, liver or shellfish.

Now on the other hand cholesterol can be too low. You don't hear about that. But that can be detrimental also. The brain is made up of mostly fat. Cholesterol is an essential component of cell membranes. A low cholesterol reading could be a signal that the necessary absorption of fats is not occurring. Without enough cholesterol one's health can also be adversely affected.

Shellfish and Liver: These two also were on the shit list for cholesterol yet they are wonderful sources of protein, iron and iodine, especially for someone with low blood sugar.

Whole grains: It is important for a carbohydrate to be as close to its original form as possible. When it is stripped of its bran it loses its nutritional value. Putting it back in the way they "fortify" a cereal with vitamins is not the same and not utilized by the body properly. Why the hell did they have to take it out in the first place? Yes Granola was a wonderful and delicious invention. It is whole grain. Just be careful of the added sugar and the hydrogenated oil in it. There are great recipes for making your own and you can control the sugar and fat that's added. Some additional hints are to eat old fashioned (not quick oats) oat meal instead of oat cereal. Have brown rice instead of white rice (it contains the original form whereas the white rice is stripped and the same as eating white bleached flour). Whole grain breads instead of the white bread.

Also consider that wheat is not the only grain on the planet. There are other grains like Quinoa, Amaranth, Rye, Buckwheat, Spelt and Kamut just to name a few.

I have a friend who goes and buys every grain imaginable from the health food store bulk bins. He mixes them up with some brown rice flour and water to bind it. He bakes them into hockey puck lumps and then he eats these for breakfast. He warned me I had to have sound dental status before partaking of one of these grainy delights. Oh my God!!! It was like chewing on a brick! I was worried about cracking a tooth. However, these little fuckers were hardy.

Veggies and Fruit: Fresh as you can get them. Organic if you can afford them. Some vegetables are better for you raw, however, some only release good nutrients if they're cooked. Cooked is OK. If you have to choose between canned and frozen, choose frozen. The canned ones are all cooked out and have added salt and things to preserve them, not to mention the can also contributes compounds into your food that is not good for the body. When things are frozen, they are picked and then parboiled and frozen right away, preserving the nutrients.

Dairy: I did not list dairy in the daily requirements. Even though dairy has good things like protein, calcium and tryptophan, we are not built to assimilate milk products after being an infant. Even then it is really only Mother's milk we are able to digest. Yes, I imagine we'd all like to stay on the tit in one way or another but I'm afraid it's pretty much not in the program. Dairy can be very high in saturated fats and cause constipation, as with cheese. Real ice cream is milk fat and other ice creams have a lot of sugar and additives. It's best to limit dairy. If you absolutely have to, then eat the Greek yogurts with no added flavors or sugars. Yes that's right, plain. Add some fresh fruit if you can't stomach straight soured milk. It does provide protein, calcium and the necessary bacteria for a healthy digestive tract (which is epidemically compromised in this society).

CALORIES

It is amazing to me we are not all schizophrenic from all the double doses of brainwashing we receive, not just daily but exponentially through the particle beam bombarding our brains through advertising. Here are the messages: "Indulge in that wicked pleasure..... you deserve it.....consume that divine piece of chocolate.....live for your taste buds.......you're privileged!!!!" "But WAIT!!...Don't get your credit card out yet,.....you get more!" The Ad reads: "Are you Fat? Got those unsightly bulges? Do you have your own zip code? Want to lose that tire around your gut? Want to stop looking like a pregnant hog stuffed into a Speedo? Want to see your dick again?....... Then go on this crash diet...take these pills.....let us inject you with God knows what that we bribed the FDA into approving even though all those lab rats died the first day....eat this special reconstituted food so you'll be dependent on us and not know how to cook for yourself.....buy this workout tape because you're too stupid to know how to go for a walk"

Are you getting the whole craziness to this? "Live for your taste buds so we can get rich, but oh darn it I'm so sorry you're a pasty lazy blob." "Do you also have social anxiety and low self esteem? And you're now getting depressed? Don't worry our cousin the pharmaceutical company has medication for you to counteract all that. Makes me think we're no different than the cattle they're fattening up on non-nutritive silage at the stockyards.

It's SIMPLE. You eat foods that jump start your

metabolism. Most of those foods are as close to their original state as possible. No, I did not say "natural."

The whole calorie counting thing is flawed because it does not take into account the quality of the food or the nutritional content of the food. You could stay on a 1,000 calorie a day diet and maybe lose weight. But those thousand calories could just be French fries and catsup. They have no nutrition in them!!! You are literally starving to death. Then your natural response will be to eat even more because your body is desperately searching for nutrients.

Let me sidetrack for a minute. A little lesson in starvation. In third world countries where food is scarce and people are actually starving to death, they are UNDERnourished. In this country we have an abundance of food, people are obese from so much consumption, but we are starving in a different way; we are MALnourished. In other words we have plenty of food with no nutrition so we suffer from deficiencies and maladies, but certainly not body mass.

OK, remember the kidney story? The body is the same way. If you starve it, it slows down the metabolism in order to conserve every calorie possible. The body has sent out the Def Con 5 alert that there is a famine. Yes, folks we are not that evolved from our cave dweller ancestors. Our bodies are still programmed to identify "a lack of natural resources". So any calorie you eat will convert to fat if you have been starving it or consuming non-nutritive foods. God forbid if you begin eating normal amounts of food or binge. You'll gain more weight than you did before.

Hey Kiddies, I've got a closet full of the T-shirts on this one. I did the starvation diets. They don't work. They set you up for being fatter and more out of shape, lethargic and unhealthy. Then you feel worse about yourself, discouraged, angry, maybe even depressed. When people ask me what my secret is for maintaining my weight I say as forceful as I can (hopefully after a Binaca blast), "EATING!!!!!" Of course I don't see any blinding light bulbs go on over their heads.....No "Ah Ha's", just an open mouth with that "Huh?" look.

Then I explain how eating is the key to boosting your metabolism. You have to shut off the famine alert and turn on the abundance awareness that it's OK to burn those calories as there is plenty of nutritious food available. (We will talk about how to burn some of those calories in a later chapter.)

So my hardcore message on Calories is this:

1. You cannot starve yourself in order to lose weight, keep it off for good and remain healthy.

2. You also cannot eat a thousand calories of chocolate fucking cake all day and lose weight, keep it off for good and remain healthy.

3. You can, however, boost your metabolism by eating foods as close to their original form as possible, thereby increasing your chances of burning up stored calories in the form of fat.

4. If you've been on a roller coaster in your lifetime with weight, then do not expect overnight results after correcting your "eating program". It will take time, patience and persistence to re-regulate your body so it will respond the way you want it to.

BLOOD SUGAR

No, needing to create and regulate your blood sugar does not mean eating sugar to do so. Yes eating sugar will convert to blood sugar but in a very dangerous way. Get this in your mindset now, otherwise don't bother reading any farther. Blood sugar has everything to do with that roller coaster you've been on. So if you don't intend to seriously give up the sugar then "see ya".

All foods create blood sugar. I wish it was called something else. Well it is…glucose. But still there is so much confusion on this because people automatically think that sugar is a necessary fuel source. It's not. Blood sugar is. It's your nutrient factor that flows through your veins and feeds all your tissues and organs. Without it you can go into a coma and die. AND, with too much you can go into a coma and die. How's that for Reality TV!!?? You're screwed no matter where that teeter totter lands, aren't you? Or like a tight rope.
But you can widen that tight rope into a nice wide path and not fall off into a bramble bush full of African bees. So here's the skinny (excuse the pun because maintaining your blood sugar can also help you lose weight)…..
When you get up in the morning your blood sugar is low

from fasting some 10 to 12 hours. Hopefully you didn't eat all the way up to midnight and then sleep walk to the Ding Dong drawer at 2 AM. That's why the morning meal is called "break…fast". You are breaking the fast. What you put in your mouth and swallow first thing in the morning (yeah, oral sex nutrients count) will affect your body's chemistry the rest of the day.

Naturally (oops I slipped), the "what" is critical. Again here's another roller coaster you could be on with the wrong choices. First of all, the enemy is insulin. When we eat a high glycemic food (go look it up) it stimulates insulin to pour into your system. Insulin spikes, using up the blood sugar in your bloodstream and then causes the blood sugar to drop lower than before you ate the high glycemic food. When the blood sugar is low it triggers cravings for more high glycemic foods. Did you feel it? You just hit the second nose dive on that roller coaster.

Insulin then converts that blood sugar into fat while also holding any stored fat at bay, preventing it from being burned up and utilized for energy. So not only can you not lose weight, you are continually adding to it. Vicious cycle. Insulin is also destructive to the cells, the veins , the organs and other hormones. Follow a Diabetic sometime. They are at risk for poor wound healing, gangrene, loss of limbs, blindness, kidney failure and erectile dysfunction, to name a few. Why? Because insulin destroys the little teeny veins called capillaries. When capillaries are weak, they rupture, releasing blood……hence blindness when the eyeball fills with blood. Not a good prognosis. But you go ahead and put that Krispy Kreme in your mouth and see what happens when you play Russian Roulette with your body.

Our bodies were not built to consume mass quantities of carbs. We predominantly ate animal flesh and only vegetation occasionally when we could find it. That vegetation which would have had some carbohydrates were not simple sugars or refined stripped grains. They were complex carbohydrates (remember in their original form) that had more protein content, took longer to digest and did not spike insulin.

Stripped Down Carbs ---Naked and Naughty:

Let's face the whole nasty truth----refined stripped down carbs (high glycemic factor) are like heroin. It is ultimately addictive, creating the insulin/blood sugar loop creating more and more need and desire for carbs and sugar.

I just go ballistic when I see these "Oh you can cheat on your diet and have that cheeseburger or hot fudge sundae and still stay on your diet". Excuse me!? Who the fuck do you think you are fooling? Really, I can? Oh Geez, silly me.
STOP!! Here's what's wrong with that message. Just from my own experience, when I have that wheat or sugar, it is the same as if I were a hardcore heroin addict standing in line down at the Methadone Clinic to get my dose. The worker says, "Oh that's OK Sweetie, you can have a little shot of heroin (hot fudge sundae) once in awhile.....you can just get right back on your program, no sweat". Like hell I can. They'd find me slobbering

incoherently on the couch after a week long binge, trails of green and brown goo drooling down my chin with the empty gallon carton of chocolate mint ice cream stuck to my lap, the test pattern all ablaze on the TV. Don't believe it for a moment folks.

Refined carbs are addicting. Plain and simple. It's the same as kicking heroin. Once you do, don't tempt fate. It's not worth it.

Here's a simple formula:

1. Break your fast with proteins. This does not release insulin, yet you are beginning to build your vital blood sugar. You may add whole grains to this as long as there is no sugar, jam, syrup or honey involved. And it cannot be cereals either unless you are absolutely certain there is no sugar, dextrose, sucrose, fructose......no "oses" added. Not even corn syrup. A bagel is refined grains, so it has a high glycemic factor and will spike insulin. No bananas, no oranges, no juices of any kind (in the AM) as these all go straight to the blood stream and release insulin immediately. (Why do you think Diabetics carry orange juice around with them? When they've had too much insulin they can counter it instantly by drinking the juice and it goes right to the blood stream to correct the imbalance.)

2. One only needs to keep snacking (remember that constant "eating thing" to boost metabolism also?) on non-insulin releasing foods until lunch

time. Things like crunchy vegetables and fruits, carrots, apples, celery, nuts, cheese, eggs…..etc.

3. Lunch is a balance of protein, vegetables and whole grains. You have now built your blood sugar to a good level. It should stay stable now since the building up part was the vulnerable time for fluctuations from insulin.

4. Snacks until dinner can now be soft fruits (oranges, bananas, peaches,…) which do have some sugar content that might release some insulin, but since the blood sugar is level it can handle it. You have made it past the roller coast stage of your day.

5. Dinner is the same as lunch.

I will warn you, though. There are a few side effects to eating like this:

a. You may have scads of energy.

b. You may not have that afternoon single cell brain slump.

c. You may lose weight.

d. You may feel good about yourself.

e. Your moods may be cheerier and stable.

f. You may sleep better at night (because that roller coaster doesn't stop just because you fell asleep. Low blood sugar will wake you up searching for food.)

g. You may not need that anti-depressant or bipolar medication anymore.

h. You may avoid developing Diabetes.

i. You might live longer.

j. Your doctor might tell you to get the fuck out of his office because your labs were so fabulous.

k. Your aches and pains may go away.

l. Your relationships might improve.

m. You may be more productive at your job.

n. You may teach your children how to eat right so they don't grow up to be on a roller coaster (unless they go to Coney Island).

Those are just a few side effects to scare you with. I believe in fear tactics.

BLOOD TYPE

Now I thought this was hokey the first time I heard about eating according to what blood type you are. But once I witnessed the results of doing so, I was convinced to try it. Now I wouldn't even consider eating a food that is not in line with my blood type, that's how valid it is to me.

Basically certain foods are not digested and assimilated properly by certain blood types. If a blood type eats a food that is not beneficial to it, it will produce toxins. The body then produces fat cells in order to warehouse these toxins. There are many other side effects that ensue also, such as fatigue, achy and swollen joints, bloatedness, bowel irregularities, weight gain, arthritis.....the list goes on.

Blood type eating is pretty easy. There are "shoulds" and there are "shouldn't" for each blood type, O, A, B and AB. If you predominantly choose from the "shoulds" list you will give yourself a greater chance of experiencing optimum health and feeling really good.

The basis behind this is again the way we ate as cave dwellers. We ate animal flesh and occasional vegetation. The vegetation back then was not wheat. So the oldest blood type going back to the cave days is "O". O's cannot handle wheat or dairy. Sorry, there's no getting around it. I'm an O. After I gave up sugar I then had the insurmountable task of giving up wheat. It was worse than the sugar. It took me 2 years of falling off the wagon to finally wake up one day and say, "Alright already, enough of this shit, I'm doin' it!!" It was one of the best things I ever did for myself.

Wheat is a newer grain in the scheme of humans being on the planet. Our systems are not built for it. Same with Type A blood. Sorry again. The only people who can handle some wheat are B's and AB's as they are a younger blood types that were around when wheat was introduced. Sometimes people's reactions to wheat are so severe it is actually a disease called Celiac. There is actually a test for it. But you don't have to have the full blown Celiac disease to experience ill effects from eating wheat.

Hence the reason corn-fed cattle is not a healthy choice. Corn is not a natural food source for cows. So cows do the same thing as human bodies do. It produces fat (marbled meat) to harbor those toxic byproducts of unnatural food. Anything else given to that animal is also stored in the fat such as antibiotics and steroids. Grasses are the natural food of cattle. So let me clarify here......Beef is a good food!!!! If cattle have been grass-fed then it is a lean healthy meat which is high in Omega 3's.

The same can be applied to farm-raised Salmon. Many of them have been fed corn. This is not the natural food for Salmon and they will respond the same way cattle do. Their fat will not contain the good Omega 3's but will contain the harmful Omega 6's. (Omega 6 is harmful when it outnumbers the content of Omega 3's). So here you are doing the right thing and eating really good fish and it's bad for you. Goddamnit!!!! And add to that, they are adding pink dye to the fish because it was raised in captivity. It is white and doesn't look like the attractive pink we have come to associate with healthy Salmon.

Some Success Stories:

There was a 70 year old woman who had arthritis in almost every joint of her body and was plagued by constant swelling and pain in those joints. Needless to say her sleep also suffered from not being able to ever get comfortable or pain free, and she also struggled with her weight. After going on the blood type diet for one month the swelling went down in all her joints, the pain went away and an unexpected loss of 22 pounds occurred without even trying.

Another lady I know took it upon herself to just stop eating wheat as she had heard me speak of it so often. (You invariably have to talk about it when you graciously decline scrumptious pasta, pizza and sandwiches made by other people with loving care for you). Again this woman was in her 70's and had experienced debilitating back pain for decades. She had many medical treatments and drugs including cortisone shots into her spine, all providing no relief for her. After one month of not eating wheat, she woke up one day and realized she was no longer in pain. If that wasn't evidence enough, she took a trip and was unable to get the non-wheat bread we O's seek out. She ended up eating some pasta and sandwiches with wheat in them and immediately had her old pain return. As soon as she got home she went back on being wheat free and the pain subsided once again.

I, too, am in this category. I struggled with weight, bloatedness, abdominal tenderness, moodiness and sugar cravings. After about 2 months not only were all my abdominal problems gone, I was better able to lose weight, I subtly noticed that all my sugar cravings were gone and I was no longer a slave to food. This was the best side effect ever. I was governed by my cravings. Each day was a battle. As soon as wheat enters my body, my cravings come back. I put on weight and I'm an ogre for days until I get myself cleaned out.

Steps to Take:
1. If you don't know your blood type, find out. There are inexpensive home kits to test your

blood or you can pay more and just have your doctor order the labwork.

2. Acquire the condensed version of foods that your blood type can have, at your local health food store or bookstore.

3. Just try it for 2 weeks. See how you feel.

FATS

Just saying the word fat starts the cringing process in everyone. Fats are actually our friend. You just have to know what kind you are getting and keep in mind ANYTHING in excess can be detrimental. (Did you know you can drink too much water or suck in too much oxygen? It can kill your brain). Let's see if we can clear fats of their bad press over the past few decades.

A Little History on Fats:
It is speculated that Neanderthals and Homo Sapiens consumed a lot of fat with their meat. If they didn't have the extra fat they would not survive the winter. Even though we are no longer running around in a loin cloth spearing whooly mammoths in the snow, I find this a significant point. If we haven't evolved that much from the rest of their diet, why would the fats be much different?

Fat has a function in our diets. There is a balance between protein, carbs and fats when it comes to working together to get the most out of the food. Fat by itself is beneficial to nerve cells. I have heard of a study where they limited a group of people on their fat intake to zero. Within a short amount of time the people increasingly became irritable and eventually became downright hostile, and even violent. I believe the reason is that fat helps to rebuild the myelin sheath around the nerve cell and when that doesn't happen you get irratic nerve function causing mood swings and other behaviors due to neurological dysfunction. Makes sense to me. Yes, fats are higher in calories but remember we blasted the myth about calories? If your metabolism is up because you are eating more of the right things then you will burn up those calories.

Fats vs. Oils:
Fats basically are solid at room temperature and are saturated, such as butter, lard, and animal fat. Oils are liquid at room temperature and are typically mono or poly unsaturated, such as olive, peanut, sunflower, safflower, and corn oil. (I'm not going to track down the chemical compound for you).

Polyunsaturated vegetable oils got a lot of air time not too long ago and how good they are for you as compared with saturated fat like butter. It then comes out that monounsaturated fats are even better for you and that the poly unsaturated oils can be unstable when heated. Polys are sunflower, safflower, and corn, while the monos are olive and peanut. (That's why peanut oil is good for frying).

Trans-Fats:
One of the reasons fats got such a raw deal is because

of what has been done to these oils. What they did was to take a nice vegetable oil and hydrogenate them. By adding hydrogen atoms to the oil molecule it allows the oil to be solid at room temperature. Now it's a fat. A Trans-Fat. This then makes all those irresistible crackers and cookies in boxes on the store shelf.

These hydrogenated oils also became known as margarine. In the introduction I gave an example advertising lies and margarine. The Ad World can legally call margarine vegetable oil which has the connotation of being good for you, right? The "mistruth" is that they don't tell you it's hydrogenated which overrides any health benefit of that nice oil.

So when you are at the market you must be mindful of reading labels. It has to say on the ingredients that the oil is hydrogenated. Once you see that then "YEEEEEEEEEENT!! WRONG ANSWER...... NEXT CONTESTANT!"

Peoples and Fats:
I witnessed people in Maryland living well into their 100's in a sleepy little town called Crisfield. These people literally fried everything in bacon fat. They also did not seem to have an obesity problem. So why is it they had such long lives?

Eskimoes used to live on seal meat and whale blubber. These people never had a clogged artery amongst them. Heart bypass surgery was unheard of (as well as diabetes). Now the unhealthy and unhappy ending to this story is that the Eskimo people were introduced to the

American diet------bleached stripped flour, processed sugar, salt and hydrogenated oils. Now they suffer from diabetes and triple bypass surgeries are performed on a daily basis. Just like the rest of us.

The combination of "trans-fats" and processed foods (all those things from boxes and packages to junk food) spells disaster. Obesity, clogged arteries, heart disease, high blood pressure, stroke and even cancer are linked to processed food consumption.

I guess I don't have to go into more detail on margarine vs. butter, do I? I like my non-wheat toast in the morning to be all slick and lubricated. I choose butter over margarine any day. But what I now do is pour olive oil straight on my toast. I figured why not? I want the butter to getting liquidy on my toast so why not just cut to the chase and use a liquid that's better for me? I did have to adjust to the taste but now I prefer it. Hell I even pour it on oatmeal and add a little salt (no sugar). People laugh at me when they see this. But I don't give a crap. I'm happy. Besides I've had people laugh at me all my life, either for my fat ass or for my unusual eating habits.

Public Eating

Because of the exposure of this heinous crime to our oils (and subsequently our health), many food establishments make it neon-sign-known that there are "zero Trans-fats used in our food." Yay! Good!

But wait.....then what fat or oil are you using? Here's something I have come to question. I didn't list it just for this reason. However, Canola Oil is a monounsaturated oil. This seems to be the one that is being used predominantly and touted as a beneficial monounsaturated oil.

So let me ask you this? What in the hell is a Canola? Have you ever met an actual Canola? How many Canolas had to die to make that bottle of oil? Have you ever stood watching the sun glisten on the wavering Canola crops? Do Canolas even waver?

Here's what I think, and I encourage you to go find out. I don't think there is such a thing as a Canola. I read some disturbing literature once that Canola oil was derived from the rapeseed plant. It is toxic. Canada won't even feed it to their cattle and throw it out. (Or sell it to us? How smart are we?) Hence the name Canada Oil condensed into Canola Oil.

And if the research comes flying back at me that it is a trusted monounsaturated oil that is sooooooo good for you, then you can be sure my rebuttal will be that I've also read that car oil is monounsaturated. I certainly won't be fryin' MY chicken in it!!!!

A NOTE ON RESEARCH: When you do research, please, please, please, find out who sponsored or paid for the research. Many times it is the drug companies or the food industries that have a big agenda at selling their products. And it is they who have conducted the research so they can sway the results to win their argument for or against something that will put money in their pocket. Why would they want you to get truthful information?

Cholesterol---Another Fat Fiend or Not?

Cholesterol!! It strikes fear in the hearts of many to hear it. Cholesterol in your food, cholesterol in your blood. Good cholesterol, bad cholesterol. What are we to think? What are we to do? Jesus God help us. Here are two things that may help shine a light:

1. Just because cholesterol is in a food doesn't mean it's bad for you. Liver, eggs and some seafoods have cholesterol. These are foods that are very good for your blood. Cholesterol is a food source just like any other fat. (Remember the cave guys eating a lot of fat to survive the winter?). Just because you eat it doesn't mean it converts to cholesterol in your blood. If you have elevated cholesterol levels I would have you examine the other foods you are eating and your lifestyle. You need to ask some hard questions:....are you eating lots of carbs, sugars and junk food?.... are you sedentary and don't have a lot of activity or exercise?.....are you overweight?.... is your life filled with stress?........do you have trouble falling asleep and/or staying asleep? If you answer yes to these then you're probably in trouble but not from the cholesterol you've eaten.

2. The misunderstanding surrounding cholesterol is this: Cholesterol by itself in the blood is a fat that wishes to repair cells. It is only when it becomes oxidized that it turns into a harmful chemical that attacks the heart. Oxidation comes

from many stressors in our lives-----chemicals, toxins, drugs, bad diet, radiation, emotions, lack of sleep, all work and no play...the list can go on. These stressors oxidize us on the inside in the same way the sun oxidizes the paint on your car.

However, cholesterol in itself needs to be looked at in a global way. The medical profession looks only at the symptom of high cholesterol. They do not look at what caused it. It is an intricate system involving the interplay of blood sugar, insulin receptors, liver processing, intestinal health, thyroid function and adrenal health, as well as an array of other hormones.

It is not OK to just treat symptoms, like high cholesterol with drugs, without asking the above questions. If you walked into your house and it was flooded, would you just run a de-humidifier 24 hours a day in every room thinking that will solve the problem? No, you would search out where the broken pipe was at and fix that first. Same with throwing drugs or remedies at a symptom expecting that to fix the problem.

Fat Free!??? Who Are You Kidding!?

Fat free sour cream. Fat free mayonnaise. Fat free ice cream. Fat free whipping cream. Don't you see the contradiction in each one of those substances? They're oxymorons. Fat-free Fat!! And I guess the food industries think we are just that----morons! Because we're the idiots who keep buying this shit. And it's shit!!! Something that is pure fat, like cream can't be fat free.

It is no longer anything that resembles cream. It has to be replaced with something. What then? Some magical substance that pretends to be fat and miraculously moves through your bowels without any ill effects? Come on people! Read the label. Do you even know what that shit is they've put in there? Just because you can't pronounce it doesn't mean it automatically goes off the "no-no" list. For all you know it's the chemical name for cyanide and laundry soap. More than likely it's all sugar and starches they've replaced the fat with. So how smart is it to not eat the fat but add one more thing onto your plate that will increase you insulin and convert everyone of those "forbidden-but-you-think-you're-getting-away-with-it" mouthfuls into fat on your ass!!!!

A Word on Fats vs. Carbs

I wouldn't say it is one or the other that must be chosen. The body requires a certain amount of both. It is important to understand the nature of each, the fat or the carb one is partaking of. I have already outlined each. Too be starved of either one can create imbalances, deficiencies, weakness and destruction of systems in the body. The correct ratio of protein, carbohydrates and fat is optimum nutrition. Moderation in all things does not mean cutting something out completely (unless you are sensitive or allergic to it.)

Big Bottom Line on Nutrition

If you want to stay healthy, have a crack at an extended life span, more success at losing weight, think properly, feel alive, and be a good example for the next generation;

here's the only way you can shop for food. (Hey if you raise your own food, then bully for you and you can bypass this section.) You can purchase your food from the produce section, the meat section and the dairy section. That's it. Everything else in between is kaka. It is dead food. It may keep you alive (for awhile) but it is costing you more than the excess money you're laying down for someone else to do the cooking for you. The only exceptions to the 3 sections above are that you can acquire some things out of the frozen section (fruits and vegetables) and the bread and cereal section--if it is absolutely whole grain and no sugars.

Every time you go to put something in your mouth (food-wise) stop and think. Think about your car. You are like your car. If you put sugar in the tank you will kill the engine. Same for you. Sugar laden non-nutritive items will progressively just stop you from running like a well oiled machine. For the most part we keep our cars on maintenance schedules-------change oil, rotate tires, tune-ups, lube jobs, etc. Your body needs a maintenance program too. It is not a diet. It is an eating program. You wouldn't think, "Gee if I just fill my car up once it will get 500,000 miles to the gallon". No, you have to keep refilling it and taking care of it. For the life of the car and for as long as you wish to be mobile. Same with your body. That one miracle diet is not going to last you a lifetime. It will damage you. It is a mindset to think of the way you will eat every single day. If it is overwhelming to you to think of a lifetime of fresh fruits and vegetables, and grass-fed meat, that you just want to go on some cinnamon-roll bender, then do like they do in AA. Just take it one day at a time. One day you will wake up and it will just be habit to reach for the right thing. You will begin to see all those wicked tempting things as poison. You would no more reach for those than you would a can of arsenic.

I know I'm harsh about this. But I want you to get it. Sometimes a jackass only needs a nudge to move in the direction you need him to go. And sometimes he needs a two by four upside the head. I can gently nudge you----or I can kick you in the ass. Your choice. Nutrition is your first line of defense if you want to change your life, your body, your brain and your future. Pills and surgery are only things that treat symptoms. Cures get at the source of the problem and nutrition is the foundation.

SUPPLEMENTS----THE NEW CONDIMENTS

There's so much hoopla about supplements it can make your head spin. One of the biggest arguments against supplements is, "If you just eat a balanced diet (ooo, there's that bad word) then you'll get all the nutrition you'll need". That sounds like sound advice. BUT WAIT!!!! My Bullshit-O-Meter just went off, ding, ding, ding, ding!!!!!!

First of all, food derives ITS nutrients from the soil. Our soil has been so depleted for decades that our raw foods cannot possibly contain ample nutrients.

Second of all, finding people who were actually eating balanced meals to begin with would be a miracle. Two biggies to overcome, don't you think?

So what are supplements? Basically I'm talking about vitamins and minerals. Now I'm not going to go over the list for you. You need to find out what you need. Everybody is different and has different needs. If I advised you to take iron because you are female and still menstruating and come to find out you have some rare thing that causes you to hang onto too much iron in your body, then I'd be advising you to poison yourself. Not going to do it.

I will, however, give you a few basics AND WHAT WORKS FOR ME:

1. We need B vitamins to build proteins. Much of our body is made up of protein. We derive B vitamins mainly from animal flesh. Amino acids are the building blocks of proteins. There are 8 essential amino acids the body cannot produce and must derive from animal flesh. Even if you choose not to eat animals, taking a pill that supplies these 8 essential amino acids still comes from an animal source. There is no sufficient vegetable source that can supply it. Sorry Vegans. I didn't make this stuff up. We are built to be carnivores. Our two front-set eyes are for binocular vision, our canine and incisor teeth for tearing flesh, and our digestive systems for digesting flesh.

2. Vitamin C is critical because Scurvy is not some rare Pirate Disease. People today still suffer from a vitamin C deficiency called

Scurvy. Also C builds the immune system. The immune system is not just responsible for fighting infection. Basically any cancer cell is just a normal cell that has mutated and is now reproducing itself. It is seen as a foreign body and the immune system will attack it. If our immune systems are up to snuff then they probably gobble up millions of cancer cells every day and we are none the wiser. This is why the ancient practice of Chinese Medicine is not about disease control, but about building the bodies energy stores so it can fight off anything unnatural on its own, the way it is programmed to do. The body is very smart if you allow it to do what it is capable of.

3. Calcium as well as its complements, Vitamin D and Magnesium, are crucial. They do so many more things than just build bones. Your body has an electrical system that requires certain electrolytes and minerals to make those critical conductions. When your body is deficient of Calcium it will rob it from the bones. It then has this free floating UNUSABLE form of Calcium flowing through your veins. It has to then deposit it and it becomes, arthritis, bone spurs, kidney stones, and so on.

Vitamin D assists the Calcium to be used by the bones. It is also proven to be the anti-aging vitamin. It helps to decrease depression as well.

A Good Rule of Thumb about Magnesium: It should be the same dosage as the Calcium.

Also a Note on Calcium: Calcium blocks the absorption of other nutrients and prescription drugs. Be aware of what you take your supplements or medications with, for instance don't wash them down with milk or even Calcium fortified orange juice. Calcium can be combined with Vitamin D and Magnesium, safely.

4. Fish Oils. Omega 3's are also the miracle supplement. They are anti-inflammatory and anti-oxidant. (Remember the oxidation inside your body from stressors?) Most of our processed foods and corn-fed beef and fish are high in Omega 6's. In themselves Omega 6's are not bad, but when they outnumber the Omega 3's they are bad. An example is that corn fed beef has a ratio of Omega 6 to Omega 3 of 20 to 1 when the acceptable level should be .2 to 1. Grass fed beef has the ratio of 1 to 30.

The breakdown of Omega 3's: There are 3 kinds ----ALA, DHA and EFA. They are all good, but it's the DHA that has the most profound effects. A daily dose of 600 mg. of DHA (so you have to read labels) will make a difference if someone has a weight problem, memory problems and chronic pain, just to name a few benefits.

5. Iron. If a woman is menstruating, typically she will need to replace lost iron. Men don't tend to lose their iron so should be cautious about iron intake. (Some men do need iron replacement, but that should be determined by lab tests.) Anemia can have several different causes. It is

best to figure out the cause and treat it, rather than just throw iron into your system. Although, I am a big fan of iron because most of us are deficient. Sometimes just feeling dragging, dizzy or listless can be symptoms of low iron in the blood. Iron is essential to the red blood cells as it helps carry oxygen. Something you can't afford to be without.

Other Beneficial Herbs and Supplements:

I encourage you to know your blood type. Here's why: there are many beneficial herbs out there you've probably heard about. Echinacea and Goldenseal for colds and the immune system. Alfalfa for "green food" and building and restoring the pituitary gland. St John's wort for depression. Yet each one of those I just mentioned are on the "no-no" list for blood type O's. Let me give you an example: I usually get anemic when I don't take regular iron. One time I purchased a new iron thinking I'd vary the brand. In about a week I had such horrible vertigo, the room was spinning as if I was drunk off my ass. I was grabbing for chairs and walls to keep myself from doing a face plant on the ground. Stupid me, I hadn't read the label, assuming it contained only iron. They had put all kinds of herbs in it to boost the effectiveness, one of the ingredients being alfalfa. I'm one of those Type O blood people who could be a canary in a mine if you give me alfalfa. Room-spinnin' vertigo, total loss of control, no coordination, because alfalfa is Kryptonite to me.

So just because something has great benefits doesn't mean everyone can take it. Also herbs and supplements can interact with prescription medicines. Know what you're taking. Research it. There are many web sites that will give you drug-herb interactions. Be educated and don't expect your doctor to know them. A pharmicist is probably a better resource on this as he's been trained in just that. But I urge you to be in charge of your own life.

Here are some additional Supplements and Herbs:

****Green Food - these can be different combos. Some of it being chlorophyll from plants. Or algae from the ocean. Or alfalfa. Or even a combination of vegetables if you don't eat enough. Packed full of good stuff is all I can say.

****Iodine or Kelp - Iodine is found in kelp, but if you have an allergy to iodine, then beware. Iodine aids the Thyroid which many of us have afflictions with and don't know it. Stress is the enemy to the thyroid among other organs and glands.

****L-Carnitine - an amino acid that assists the healing process.

****L-Argininine - an amino acid that improves blood circulation.

****L-Taurine - an amino acid that helps energy.

****Alpha Lipoic Acid - also helps with healing.

****Chromium - a mineral that assists with glucose utilization.

****Garlic - an antibacterial agent that works like a miracle drug for purifying mucus membranes. Also lowers blood pressure.

****St. John's Wort - an herb that can act as an anti-depressant.

****Echinacea and Goldenseal - good for the immune system.

Note: The last 3 herbs (St. John's wort, Echinacea and Goldenseal are all advised to NOT be taken by blood type "O". This is why it is beneficial to know your blood type.

Some Supplement Interactions:

++++Calcium blocks other supplements from being absorbed, especially Iron. It also can block your prescription drugs from being absorbed properly and you may not get the benefit from the drug. You may further think your drug is not working and so your doctor may increase the dosage, giving you a toxic level. So do you see how being informed could improve health but may even save your life?

++++Vitamin C negates Ginseng.

++++Vitamin C helps the absorption of Iron.

++++Calcium is best served when Magnesium equals or exceeds the dosage of Calcium.

++++Vitamin D is more effective if taken with a fatty meal.

++++Fat Soluble Vitamins are A, D, E and K. (They

are absorbed by your fat cells and stay in the body longer, so it is easier to overdose these vitamins.)

++++Water Soluble Vitamins are B and C. These flush through your body quickly.

The "RULE" with Vitamins, Herbs or Supplements - "If a little is good, a lot is not better". It is better to be conservative than to overdo those vitamins. I don't go anywhere without my stash of vitamins, However I do not jump on every band wagon that promises this is the miracle cure supplement. I'm really cautious just because that's my nature. If that wasn't enough, being highly sensitive has taught me even more caution.

Here's My Home Remedy Arsenal:

If you pay attention to the signs out there, you'll realize that bacterias, viruses and fungus are getting smarter and stronger than any antibiotics they can develop. That's because it is their nature to identify the enemy and mutate to it. Or in other words they can be bitten by a poisonous snake and develop anti-toxin to it. The more antibiotics we develop the smarter they will get.

The other thing people should know is that antibiotics only work on bacteria. You cannot kill a virus. The one thing you can do to protect yourself is to use prevention. Your immune system is a very intelligent protective shield. That is, if you take care of it. If you keep your immune system strong it will gobble up all those nasties, even cancer cells. That's its function. It is your military force in your body. It sees an enemy and it attacks it. There are swarms of horrible germs as well as beneficial germs all over and inside your body. Once your immunity goes down they attack the host (that's you). Simple. We probably all have cancer cells (which is a regular cell that mutated) that get gobbled up daily and we don't even know about it.

But if you do get sick and want to arm yourself at home, you can. The number one thing I keep on hand is Colloidal Silver. It is ionized silver in water. Its mechanism is that it disengages the breathing mechanism of bacteria and viruses. Boom. They can't build any tolerance to it and you don't have to worry about toxicity. Colloidal silver has gotten a bad rep and it's all hype. Who do you think put out the information? Go research it and find out who's behind it. Sickness is big business in our society, so why would they want you to get healthy? The only thing that could happen is your skin could get a blue tinge to it------YEAH, IF YOU DRINK 5 GALLONS OF IT A DAY!!!!!!!! You only drink a ½ a teaspoon at a time diluted in water.

The other thing I keep on hand is Grapefruit Seed Extract. Very potent and should be diluted in water. DO NOT TAKE IT STRAIGHT. It will burn your mouth. But I clean everything with it-----my fruits and veggies, my bathtub, my drinking water, my feet and my snatch. Yes it is good for yeast destruction as it eliminates bacteria, viruses and fungus. (Yeast is a fungus).

My other number one thing is Garlic. As soon as I get any respiratory thing going on I am eating raw garlic. It will purify the bugs right out of the mucus lining in your nose, throat, lungs. This is the shit!!!!

Olive Leaf Extract. Look this one up folks. You think there are no cures in this world. This one will clean out your liver and also clean out bugs that have embedded themselves into the nerve track.

Elderberry. Good to support your healing when you get flus, colds and respiratory infections.

Oreganocillin. This is a combination that will clean out the residual stuff after you've suffered from a bad respiratory infection and have that lingering cough and general not well feeling.

Honey. Good for inside and out. If you suffer seasonal allergies it is advised to get locally grown honey as the bees have infused the honey with the pollens you are reacting to. It is a form of an allergy shot. You will eventually build up a tolerance if you are exposed to the things you are allergic to. On the skin it is healing whether it is for skin care or even wound care. (Note: Never give honey to babies).

In Summary:

Supplements are just that. They are an addition to the other things that you are doing for your health. Supplements will not save you if you are living on processed shit food. But they will complement nutritious foods in a more pronounced way. Remember that your health is like a wheel. Everything you do (or don't do) are the spokes in the wheel. Each one contributes to the wheel's ability to stay fully round and able to roll. Supplements are just one spoke.

CHAPTER 4: ELIMINATION
OR
"SHIT MUST HAPPEN"

I'm now appealing to all the assholes out there. The subject most people avoid like it doesn't matter. Well whatever goes in must come out. This is very important.

Bottom line----if you're not going regularly then you have waste products sitting in your intestines, fermenting and being re-absorbed into your system. That would be like taking a shit in the toilet, not flushing and then going back into the bathroom and filling up your teapot with toilet water to brew your chamomile tea. How refreshing. NOT!!!!

It not only will make you toxic, it will start to expand the colon, break it down and then become impacted. This means it becomes so hard it will not move and becomes a medical emergency. The Emergency Rooms see this every day where they have to dig out someone's shit for them.

Just like your muscles with weight lifting, your fingers

with piano lessons and your brain with math problems, your bowels can be trained also. And need to be. A wise OB-Gyn MD friend once told all his patients, "heed to the need to purge". When you feel that urge, GO! Even if you don't feel it, then you need to schedule a daily time to sit and have it move. It is actually called bowel training. It responds.

If you are having trouble going, then you may need more fiber. Water is also crucial to having a movement. Without enough water, any fiber in the fecal mass will draw water out of you. This will in turn cause you to be more dehydrated, causing a vicious circle of water deficiency compounding the constipation even more. Laxatives, however necessary in dire moments, are not something one should rely on regularly. Laxatives make the bowel dependent on them. They break down the natural structures and tone of the bowel making them less efficient to move along the poop. Thus more dependency on the laxative to get things moving.

Now the opposite can be true also. Many people suffer from loose bowels. They are possibly not able to absorb enough nutrients out of their food because of this and they are losing vital fluids. There could be many reasons why this is happening. This too needs investigating. I'm not for plugging it up with medication, however if it is severe it does need to be controlled. Nutrition is always a good place to start. It could be a mild food sensitivity as in the blood type diets or regular plain old food allergy. You need to find the reason why it's happening.

There are four main ways the body eliminates waste products.

1. The Bowels eliminate the food you've eaten after extracting the nutrients.

2. The Kidneys filter all your blood and remove waste products and fluid regulation.

3. The Skin protects you from any germs entering body but releases fluid for cooling and releasing toxins and electrolytes.

4. The Lungs take in oxygen and put it into the blood then exchanges out the carbon dioxide waste from your blood and releases that CO2 out your lungs. Your lungs also release a lot of fluid. (Something to keep in mind during hot days or during exertion.)

All these systems need plenty of water as all of them release water. We must replenish water constantly.

Elimination is simple, so I don't need to dwell on it, do I? Oh sure I could go into all the color, size, shape and even smell of it. If it floats or sinks. But I'll leave that up to you. All those things have meaning. Deal with your own shit, OK? Understand your shit. You're responsible for your own shit so keep your shit together.....hopefully in the toilet where it belongs and not rotting in your bowels.

CHAPTER 5: EXERCISE
OR
"MOVE YOUR ASS"

If you don't move your ass, the sooner you're part of the grass. Let's not even harp on the fact that decade after decade Americans have become obese cows. Hell, cows are trimmer than we are. Set the fact aside that losing weight depends on movement of some kind. What I'm talking about is that your life actually depends on movement.

Without activity and yes, the four letter word "exercise ", the body does not produce the blood chemicals that keep the heart strong and vibrant.

Without activity there is no resistance that keeps bones replacing bone mass and remaining dense and strong.

Without activity the blood doesn't circulate, deliver oxygen or keep the vessels open and pliable.

Without activity a body loses balance and coordination.

Without activity the inner brain shrinks.

Without activity the body/brain does not produce the "feel good" hormones that can fight depression, fatigue and even pain.

Without activity the muscles atrophy, losing good enzymes that benefit many systems and also decrease the metabolism (your steam engine).

There is so much that depends on your activity level. Without activity the body basically becomes weak, uncoordinated, high risk, fragile and non-vital.

So let's look at what exercise does. It builds muscle, which is what determines how hot our metabolism burns the calories we've consumed or stored as fat. When people starve themselves they digest muscle first because it's easier to digest than fat. So now there's less muscle. When we do start to eat again, and we will, then the metabolism is slower and will convert those calories right to fat.

There are two kinds of exercise needed. 1) Aerobic or Cardio workouts. 2) Weight training. Aerobic is the sustained movement that keeps your heart pumping at an increased level for 12 minutes or longer (not including the warm-up and cool down periods). The heart rate cannot be maxed out though, otherwise it becomes and anaerobic (without oxygen) exercise and creates an entirely different response in the body. With sustained moderate heart rate increase a body releases those wonderful enzymes that are good for the heart and also will increase the metabolism to continue to burn fat even after the exercise is over. Anything like fast walking, bicycling, dancing, stair stepping, treadmills, swimming, can all be aerobic. In weight lifting the body builds muscle which also supports bones and bone density, coordination and increasing metabolism. It does not require bench pressing 200 pounds and being able to clean and jerk 500 pounds. Repetition with minimal weights will eventually feel like 100 pounds. If you do 20 reps of 3 pounds with your arms, believe me you will feel "the burn."

The mistake most people do is to overdo. Any exercise regime must start off slow and not to excess, especially if one is out of shape and not used to activity of this nature. The hardest thing to do is to be patient and persistent. You cannot get overnight results. The body must adjust to fitness program of any kind. It takes time to shed those fat pads. Anything that happens quickly is probably not fat, but more likely muscle and water. Besides, if you overdo it and get really sore, you probably won't go work out for a week. Then one week turns into two, three…..then those éclairs are starting to look real good because now you're frustrated again, and maybe even depressed and need to stuff those feelings of inadequacy. So you gotta do the AA of Fat-Aholics 12 step thingy…."one day at a time" and try not to get too anxious with the results. Keep at it. A little each day. It doesn't take much. Before you know it, you may even be addicted to the "happy juice" your brain is secreting and want to exercise all the time.

If you want to buy fancy work out equipment, God

only knows I've thrown away good money on them, then so be it. Some of them are actually pretty good. Or if you need to make a commitment to a gym and pay the monthly price, then by all means, great, do it. Sometimes it's good to hire a one-time personal trainer to show you how to do things right so you won't hurt yourself, to set goals, and have someone to answer to. Find out what time works best for you. I find that if I don't fall out of bed and onto the equipment and just get it over with, I will never do it later in the day. Also I do it that way because when the blood sugar is low in the morning it's best for fat burning to work out at that time. It forces the body to burn the fat since there's not a lot of blood sugar available. But if night time is the right time, then there you go. Everyone has different times of the day when they are at their best. It's their natural biorhythms. Mine is in the morning. Then I go to shit by the afternoon.

Find something you love to do. I happen to love music. If music is on I don't have to think twice about what to do. My body just wants to move, even on my most sluggish days. You don't need any special aerobics class to show you how to move. Any movement, remember? If you love your dog, take him for a run. Being sedentary is not good for him either, so he will benefit from your time together. If you love to shop, go to the mall and power walk around the place a few laps and then allow yourself to shop afterward. Hell if you're angry all the time get a damn punching bag and hit the sucker for half an hour. You'll get in shape and the side effect will be you probably won't be biting off everyone's heads anymore because you'll feel calmer. Whatever it is you like you can find a way to make an exercise out of it.

There is one thing I need to insist on. Always warm up before any exercise. The muscles need to warm up, the tendons and ligaments need to stretch. You can damage those things if you start sprinting or jerking weights around without limbering up. I'm sure even those thoroughbred race horses get a good warm up and rub down before a race. Also, if you're ever too out of breath to talk or continue, you need to slow down or even stop. If you feel any severe pain, especially in your chest, please stop or get help. "No pain, no gain" is not necessarily correct. Exercise should not be painful. Better to do too little than too much.

The infamous, "They", have proven that exercise, at any age, is beneficial and produces results. There was a study done on folks in a convalescent hospital who had been bed bound and could not even stand up on their own feet anymore. Starting with a slow and careful regime, these people were all eventually out of bed, walking and doing exercises. They had regained their muscle tone, balance and coordination.

This last story tells us that it is never too late to become active and reverse the effects of non movement. If these old folks can get out of their wheelchairs, then you can too. One of the excuses that drives me crazy is, "I have bad knees and I'm in too much pain to walk." Yet when I'm looking at the person they are over 250 pounds at least. The part about this that messes with my brain is that I bet their knees wouldn't hurt if they did not weigh so much. Yet I'm sure they are in so much pain now they cannot walk. Now I cycle back into my exercise archives that a side effect of proper activity can reduce pain. So my prescription is still exercise. Almost all of us resist discipline. It's something that needs to be done just like any other maintenance regiment whether for your car, your house or your body. Move. Move anything. If you are in bed, a wheelchair or a ride-about-cart, move your arms. Scrunch your butt muscles. Isometrics. Aerobics can be done in a sitting position until you are strong enough to stand up. It can be done. So do it.

Chapter 6: Sleep - Now,
Not When You're Dead

Sleep now or forever hold your piece of paper with the fucked up numbers on your lab test results, your blood sugar or your blood pressure. Lack of sleep takes years off your life.

We do not value sleep in this society. And we especially don't value just resting or taking naps. Sleep is the red-headed step-child. Work, work, work. Go, go, go. Do, do, do. Push, push, push. But God forbid don't just sit down and rest for a minute.
Or be quiet, with no distractions, and think your own thoughts. Scary.

Sleep perchance to dream. What an elusive concept both things are. Sleeping and dreaming. Yet both so vital, so necessary for your brain. Everything is dependent on your brain. Your brain is the Michelin tires of your existence.....everything is riding on it. Without sleep and dreaming the brain can not revitalize itself, repair itself, refresh and rejuvenate. Studies have proven that a sleep-deprived person will have a psychotic break..... sometimes with irreparable damage. A person who abruptly stops drinking alcohol or taking barbiturates after prolonged abuse will go into D.T.s, "delirium tremens," which is a medical emergency. The alcohol and the barbiturates suppress the dream state. Therefore the brain is "starving" for the dream cycle. When the drug is stopped the brain goes into a frenzied dream state similar to hallucinations, only worse. The entire body is at risk now....all from a lack of proper brain health due to abnormal sleep and deficient dreaming. Odd. Fragile but formidable.

Let's go on to add that studies have also linked obesity, diabetes and alzheimers (to name a few again) to deficient sleep. The brain is an intricate enigma full of neurons, with chemicals that conduct the electrical current between them called neurotransmitters. The brain is responsible for signalling glands to emit hormones that regulate everything in your body from urine output/retention, to menstrual cycles, to fight or flight response, to glucose consumption, to emotions. It is a symphony filled with mystery and genius. Would you really want to throw a monkey wrench into the orchestra pit? Why then would you tamper with your brain by depriving it, let alone inducing it, with some toxic chemicals of your own choosing. (I'll leave the identification of those chemicals up to you, whether it is artificial sweeteners to tobacco to street drugs, or the entire gamut in between).

First, you must be able to fall asleep. Sounds simple, right? If you're fortunate enough to be one of those people who have a tight relationship with the Sand Man, then talk to someone who doesn't. They'll describe things like insanity, hell, the wailing and gnashing of teeth when that elusive somnolence evades them for hours on end. Once that occurs the next challenge is to remain asleep for a good stretch of time. There are several layers of sleep that allow the brain to heal and repair itself. If it is interrupted it has to start all over again. The clock is ticking and it can't ever recapture that cycle again. The hours of the day have an effect on the chemicals and state of the brain. You can't fool it.

The other component is the dream state. A most beneficial yet mysterious activity of the brain. Within those cycles and layers of sleep the dreaming patterns are allowed to occur. If you don't get to those dream states, regardless of whether you remember any of them or not, it will affect your health. It will also affect mood and energy levels. It could cause a real deficit in ability to physically and mentally function. For example, driving while sleep-deprived is equated to driving while under the influence of alcohol.

To go one step further on the proof of the importance of dreaming, when a person consumes years of alcohol or barbiturates, the dream state is severely halted. When the alcohol or barbiturates are abruptly stopped the brain is so starved for the dream state it will violently jump right into the dreaming, causing hallucinations and D. T.'s   This is actually a medical emergency and can cause seizures, coma and death if not monitored by the medical profession. I'd say that's pretty good evidence that dreaming is essential.

Now the opposite of not getting enough sleep is too much inactivity. Being sedentary. I feel I must mention this here as it comes back to balance. We are striving for healthy, restful sleep, with proper dream time. Yet, we don't want to negate our need for healthy activity by becoming overly focused on resting. This society tends to take something beneficial and run with it to extremes, so I don't want this need to sleep to be one of those.

So if there is a sleep problem in your life, there are many ways to go about solving it. I won't promise you it's easy or quick. The answer is not a pill, which is cheating and creates bad sleeping patterns. Particularly if you wake up naked on the highway after taking a sleep aid. The answer is good habits. Just like any other training you have to commit to doing things that are a regimen. It's called "sleep hygiene". Beginning to prepare yourself for sleep at the same time each night. Turning off the TV or computer. Brush your teeth, take warm baths, write lists so you won't obsess about shit all night. Is the bed and pillow right for you? Do you need to prop yourself up? Is the room temperature right? Do you need white noise or soft music in the background? Is your blood sugar under control, because low blood sugar will wake you up in the middle of the night. Is your thyroid under control? This will disturb sleep also. Did you drink too much fluid before bed and will have to take a leak several times? Did you keep your caffeine to a minimum? This includes coffee, tea, sodas, chocolate. Caffeine is contained in many things. There are many good meditation tapes out there for sleep. They are worth investigating.

Things to ask yourself concerning sleep:

1. What time do you try to attempt sleep? The hours before midnight have a greater impact on the quality of sleep than all the hours you can possibly sleep in in the morning. There is a thing called the circadium rhythm that your body adheres to and if you go against the timing of it, it can kick you in the ass.

2. Do you fall asleep easily? If yes great. If not see all my suggestions above.

3. Do you stay alseep? Getting up all hours of the night will mess up the release of Melatonin, the sleep hormone. Melatonin is released at certain times and if your eyes are exposed to any light during the night it disrupts the effects and you have to start all over.

In other words, Melatonin must build up in your system during the day. It's what makes you drop off to sleep. Once the sleep is disrupted, the Melatonin cannot be replenished just like that. So you're kinda screwed once it gets disrupted.

1. Do you snore? This hinders oxygen to the brain and the many health and mood issues I've mentioned can occur.

2. Do you stop breathing all together? Sleep apnea is a serious condition. This really deprives the brain of oxygen and can be life threatening. If

you suspect you have this or the person you share a bed with knows you do this, I highly recommend you go have a sleep study done. They will monitor you all night and even check your oxygen level when the breathing stops. There is help for apnea and it needs to be addressed.

3. Do you allow yourself naps? These are powerful regenerators.

4. Have you kept your stimulant consumption to a minimum during the day? Caffeine can stay in the body for a good portion of a day, lasting well into the night.

5. Do you have nightmares or PTSD? If you do, get help. Therapies that assist in minimizing or alleviating the cellular memory of trauma will significantly help your sleep, as well as your life.

6. Do you know your blood sugar levels or your blood pressure? Diet has a significant effect on sleep.

7. Do you know the condition of your thyroid? This is compromised in many people who don't even know it. It affects sleep as well as metabolism, energy, skin, hair, bowels and even emotions like depression. It is known that chronic stress levels release cortisol, which in turn takes a toll on the thyroid gland. (Not to mention putting fat deposits in the belly region, which is not good for the heart).

Nurse Rattschidt

OK, so I've given you enough to think about that you'll probably lose sleep over it. Write down your concerns so you can forget about it and just get a good nights sleep. Oh and it helps if you have someone to tuck you in, read you a bedtime story, look under the bed for the monsters, and kiss you goodnight.

CHAPTER 7: PSYCHO-ILLOGICAL ISSUES
OR
"ARE YOU MENTAL?"

I heard something long ago that I thought applied to a lot of people, including myself. A card that read "I'm tempermental.......10% temper and 90% mental." Perfect. Sounds funny but it's the truth. There's no escaping the fact that our thoughts are things. Or to put it the way Einstein coined it "E= MC squared." This means that something as intangible and the equivalent of air can manifest itself into something real and solid. Your thoughts and emotions manifest into reality at every moment whether you are aware of it or not. Whether you want to admit it or deny it, it happens.

A perfect illustration is the concept of impending threat. The mind recognizes danger. Way back when it was a saber- toothed tiger on your ass.......your adrenals pumped out adrenaline causing you to shit and run. It shuts down all functions that can temporarily take a back seat to harnessing all your ability to run as fast as you can and get the fuck out of there. It's called fight or flight. Yet now in our society, we are in a constant state of fight or flight just in our daily work lives.....gotta get the kids to soccer practice, gotta get that progress report to the Boss by five, gotta get to the dentist on time and I'm stuck in traffic, "mother fucker cut me off!!!!!!" Our bodies were not meant to sustain this kind of constant angst and they pay dearly for it. The cortisol gets released to counter the adrenaline. That in turn spikes our insulin, causing cravings. We stuff our faces with comfort food to numb ourselves. This causes insulin to surge and convert those meaningless calories right to belly fat. It puts demands on our hearts to feed that fat with blood. Our blood pressure goes up. Our brains are starving. Our veins are hardening. And it's a vicious cycle spiralling us downward right into the devil's waiting arms.

So do you still think thoughts are not things? How do we manage that? It's not like you can get ahold of it and remold it like a lump of clay. Yet it's powerful and sometimes all-consuming. The drug companies have made billions on the pills they are pumping into us for our thoughts, our moods, our sleeplessness even our shyness. Do you really think there's a magic pill? Well you can certainly take them and anesthetize yourself, but it doesn't take away any problems. It's like taking all your bills and throwing them in the garbage. You don't see them anymore but you still owe.

Face it, no one gets off the planet without getting bashed in one way or another. Very few people I've met have led idyllic lives. Abuse and trauma come in many forms. It leaves its mark on the brain, the mind, the spirit, the body, right down to the cellular level. It has to be addressed just as an infection must be dealt with. You wouldn't let an infection in your body go untreated until it festered and became gangrenous, would you? This is the same thing only in an elusive intangible form.

The difficult part about our psyche is that it requires unique individualized approaches to solving the issues that haunt us. I'm certain I will have to cover it in another book because every single person is different and responds differently to a myriad of approaches.

You can cover all the other bases in your life that we've already gone over, diet, exercise, the whole nine yards.....but if you do not have a handle on your "inner environment" then your outer environment will certainly go to shit. This could manifest in so many ways, like a messy house, can't follow through on anything, bad bosses, bad jobs, bad relationships, car accidents, physical aches and pains, frequent illnesses, poor finances.......the list goes on. As a matter of fact, if you did do everything right for your health except deal with your psychological issues, it would be the same as buying only the most nutritious organically grown foods and cooking them in sewer water. Your mind, your emotions are the very foundation on which your health and the outcome of your life depend on.

An extension of your mind-set would also include your spiritual connection. How you relate to some higher power than yourself. Whether it be religious or not, it doesn't matter what or who you call it. Something greater than yourself that gives you a sense of right or wrong. A sense of belonging. Guidance and comfort. Love. Inspiration, purpose and your own evolution. Here again, there could be six billion religions because each person has their own way of relating to this. It does not require anyone else to tell you how to do it. It is a unique relationship between you and the Universe, Father Sky, Buddha, Jesus or a Guardian Angel. Whatever. I can't list six billion ways. I've even heard that our ancestors and loved ones wish to speak to us and help us if we could just open ourselves up and listen.

A last word on abuse.....Abuse does not equal Excuse! I am livid every time I hear of a court case where the defense is "I couldn't help but hack up, rape and strangle that little girl because I was abused." Bullshit!!! By that logic, all Jews who survived the Holocaust have a right to be serial killers. These people were tragically tortured and massacred, but you don't hear about them mutilating and killing other people! Think of the other cultures who were badly mistreated and wiped out. Do they typically become criminal sex offenders? No. There is help on every corner and there is NO EXCUSE for mistreating anyone else. That's predatory behavior under the disguise of being a victim.

OK, you got all the bad head-case news, let's balance that out. On the flip side of all your mental shit, it is imperative to have enjoyment in your life. (Hopefully your brand of pleasure isn't doing heinous things to little kids). Enjoyment that is personal to you and doesn't violate the rights or well-being of another person.

What do you do for fun? What gives you passion? Motivates or inspires you? Do you have hobbies? Do you have anything you love to do and just lose track of time while you're doing it? These things are the tonic for your mental state. That saying, "all work and no play makes Jack a dull boy" is so true. However I think Jack actually gets a whole lot more than just "dull" without fun, he probably gets downright mean and maybe even sick.

Being too busy to have enjoyment is the same as being too tired to exercise. You have to carve out time for fun and your busy schedule may even improve. You have to muster the effort to work out and then your energy level will increase. I never promised you this shit would be easy.....I just told you how it works. You can make excuses not to do anything I've told you and that's up to you. But if you're one of those people who bitches and moans and complains about your life and you don't make any effort to change it, then you are going to find that you have less ears available to you over time. It's OK to whine and complain until you get over it and then are ready to do something about it. But being invested in being ill so you constantly have sympathy from other people makes me direct you back to the beginning of this chapter. Deal with your shit!!

CHAPTER 8: METAPHORMULARY

OR

"BODY LANGUAGE"

The body talks to us all the time. Our symptoms are our clues as to what's going on. You must be your body's detective because it is telling you what it needs. It's a shame that in this society we medicate away the symptoms. That's like going to a crime scene with a cleaning crew before you've documented any of the evidence or fingerprints.

Remember E=MC2? Energy equals matter? Thoughts are things? We need to be cognizant of our self-talk. What kinds of things spew out of your mouth? "I'm so pissed off!" "I could've just died." " What a pain in the ass/neck he is." "I can't stomach this anymore." Do you have problems with your bladder? Do you have any chronic ailments? Do you have back or neck pain? Do you get ulcers? It could be the chicken and the egg too. What if you aren't looking at a problem and you subconsciously keep repeating these things because deep down they're happening inside your body? Do you cause them with your persistent thoughts or is your body trying to get your attention? Things to ask yourself.

So let's look at one of the number one messengers..... pain. It's a warning. If someone came running up to you yelling and screaming that your child was in trouble, would you tackle them and then bind and gag them so it wouldn't be so? Your rationale being, "if you didn't hear it then you can rest assured your child was safe." I don't think so. Ignoring pain can be dangerous.

Pain is telling you there is a problem. It's up to you to solve it. Hopefully, if you depend on the medical profession, you have a doctor who will listen to you and not just prescribe pills to shut up that messenger. It is your body. You do not need a medical degree to know what it needs. If you are paying attention you can figure it out.

Alright, let's do some investigating. Let's look at some obvious symptoms. As you observe these keep in mind: Is there pain? Where is it? On scale of 0 - 10 (10 being worst) what number is it? What is the quality... dull, sharp, stabbing, radiating, burning, constant, once in awhile? When did it start? What were you doing or eating at the time? Here we go:

1. Headaches

2. Shortness of Breath

3. Vertigo

4. Constipation/ Diarrhea.

5. Low Energy/ Tired.

plagues wiped out entire populations. We have the same thing going on here only it's happening more slowly and silently, so no one's alarms are going off. We don't have dead people dropping in the streets with oozing sores all over their bodies. However we have people who are becoming the walking almost dead with internal sores and conditions. Obesity, heart disease and diabetes are at the top of the list.

These, to me, are the end result of what seems to be a different form of plague in itself. The "Influentia " or the force that is influencing us as a whole. TV, with its adds to eat, eat, eat!!! Drug companies and a pill for every single little ache and pain or minor discomfort, be it mental, emotional or physical. Government that will pay you to sit on your ass, be a drug addict and collect a check. The society that says, "Oh if it feels good just do it.....here pay for it with a credit card because even if you haven't worked for it you deserve it.....buy, buy, buy, eat, eat, eat, medicate, medicate, medicate!" "Don't worry about your children or your grandchildren or even the earth, just indulge and fuck responsibility to anyone, except your own comfort level."

Yet while we couch surf on our butt-boards zoning in front of the blue tube of the TV or the computer absorbing all that programming bullshit, there are even more insidious plagues that are growing that have the medical world scratching their enormous heads and creating new names for things they don't understand. Things like Fibromyalgia, Lupus, Epstein Barr, Chronic Fatigue Syndrome. These are euphemisms for "I feel like shit!" And if you translated the medical terminology for all these so-called diseases it's Latin for the doctors saying, "We don't fucking know what it is"!

Well just as you guessed, I have some theories.

PPPMMMSSSSSSS. Since PMS became passé they keep adding letters to describe how much more of a bitch she can become before her period. Yeah I know you're really not going to like me now, but I really don't give a crap. PMS is a poor excuse for bad behavior. Unless you've got real endometriosis, a tumor the size of a grapefruit in your uterus or a ruptured ovary,I don't want to hear women saying "Oh I'm PMSing so watch out!" That's saying, "I've been given an excuse to just be a total cunt and I'm runnin' with it Dude". Yeah, I said the "C" word, but if the tampax fits, wear it. Got news for you girls (and guys).....PMS is completely preventable. Proper nutrition, supplements, water, exercise and meditation will alleviate all that bloating, cramping and nasty attitude. Most women are also deficient in progesterone which is instrumental in keeping everything operating smoothly all over your body. (Now that's "hormone 101" in a nutshell.) Even if you are uncomfortable and your clothes don't fit right for a week or two, that is no reason to treat everyone like shit. They don't deserve that. (And if they do deserve it, why are you with them? Oh I forgot that's in my next book. Sorry, got ahead of myself.)

So while we're on the subject of silent epidemics and theories, here's some more for you to be judge and jury on. There is much controversy over this, but it bears mentioning. There is good evidence there is a yeast epidemic. I don't just mean a squirt of micanozole up your coochie and you're good to go kind of yeast infection. I mean candida yeast flourishing and flowing through your veins. A systemic infection.

Here's the evidence that holds water for me:

1. Antibiotics are known for killing good bacteria in your intestines causing yeast (bad bacteria) to take over and propagate in the bowel. When its numbers become so great, it begins to find its way into the blood stream and create all kinds of havoc.

2. We don't value the good bacteria in this country when we do prescribe antibiotics. In other countries it is standard to prescribe lactobacillus/ bifidus (the good bacterias found in yogurt culture) along with the antibiotic to counter the ill effects right from the start. Yes, you could eat yogurt on your own and that is a worthy effort, but consider that the sugar in the yogurt feeds the yeast. That could be counter productive. They do sell the active bacterias at the health food stores, which would be a better choice.

3. We have thrown gasoline on the fire when we feed our livestock antibiotics as well. It is no different for them. Good bacteria dies and the bad bacteria prevails and finds its way into the meat. Not to mention you are getting an extra dose of antibiotics-a double whammy!

4. Here's where havoc really sets in. Yeast in your system is that Little Shop of Horrors plant screaming, "Feed me Seymour!" Yeast craves sugars. It's a monster. Sugars come in the form of all sugars, starches and alcohol. The yeast grows and wants even more. Now you've got insulin spiking from the sugar/carb intake and the blood sugar in your body is on an endless roller coaster. This creates weight gain on top of it all. If the yeast is really severe, it sets up the body to start to attack itself due to foreign body invasion response. Hence the auto-immune diseases such as Fibromyalgia or Rheumatoid arthritis. Now there is joint pain or general pain all over the body.

5. Now a person finds himself/herself at the doctor's office in pain and wanting relief. The doctor typically only knows to medicate the pain away. So now the body (mainly the liver) has to break down and dispose of chemicals. These free float into the cells along with the yeast and why wouldn't a body be in pain with all this toxicity? The pain is worse so now the doctor gives steroids out of desperation. This may have some relief but the price is high on this one. This medication masks infection and starts to leach calcium out of your bones, not to mention other nasty things it does. If you thought your bones hurt before, have the calcium start to leave them and you'll really have something to complain about, not to mention having very brittle bones.

Do you see how this is a cascade of disaster? Just a simple cleansing and diet change could prevent all this.

A Note on Systemic Infections:

If a virus or bacteria reproduces to the point of entering the bloodstream, this is called a systemic infection. In the bloodstream it now spreads throughout the body, infecting the entire body. Some bacteria are so virile that once they reach this level they can shut down the body systems rapidly, sometimes within hours. Even with today's advanced technology and medicine, we have people die of bacterial pneumonia.

To elaborate further, we have destroyed our intestinal tracts with the antibiotics, high gluten goods, and a myriad of other offenders to the bowel. In short, we have "leaky gut" syndrome. The intestines have become broken down and allow bacteria, viruses, parasites and fungus to pass into out bloodstreams. Our body's immune system goes into high alert to attack these foreign bodies. However, we do not repair the intestines nor do we kill off the microbes present in the bowel, which continue to enter our bloodstreams. The immune system cannot shut off. It begins to attack the healthy parts of our bodies, now creating an "auto-immune" disease.

More Body Language

OK, so your body is trying to communicate with you. Let's take a look at some of those symptoms again, only from a different perspective. Let's try to rule in or out where they may have stemmed from.

Health 101: Rated R

A. FOOD

How do you feel after you eat certain things? Do you have:

1. Stomach aches
2. Heartburn
3. Bloated
4. Headaches/Migraines
5. Moody
6. Foggy
7. Joint pain
8. Constipation
9. Diarrhea
10. Weight/ Water gain

It may take some trial and error to single out the offender if it is food. Many people have low grade allergies to food and don't know it. Any one of those symptoms above could indicate a food sensitivity. There is a real basic way of getting an idea if you are sensitive to something. Take your pulse when you haven't eaten anything, like in the morning so it is your baseline reading. Something as close to your normal pulse rate as possible. Eat only one thing then take your pulse again in about 20 minutes. If your pulse has increased by 10 to 20 beats you may have a sensitivity. I can tell now when I've eaten something that is not in my best interest. Type "O" blood is not supposed to eat peanuts. I love peanuts. But in about 20 minutes after eating peanut butter my heart is pounding and about 20 beats faster. It takes a couple hours for it to return to normal. I really notice it now and it's uncomfortable not to mention it is a reminder to me that my body is saying, "hey you! Yeah you with the weak will....don't put that in your mouth anymore, got it!?"

B. ENVIRONMENT

What's in the atmosphere around you? Are there smells from chemicals or people's perfumes? Could there be molds in the building? Carbon monoxide or radon? Are you near any large electrical plants? What is the quality of the water you drink? Are you under flourescent lights all day? Do you get any fresh air?

If you are exposed to these environmental offenders you could have:

1. Headaches

2. Migraines

3. Vertigo

4. Lethargy

5. Fatigue

6. Fogginess

7. Blurred vision

8. Insomnia

9. Nausea

10. Flu-like symptoms

People can be asked to not wear perfume to work. Chemicals can be removed or cleaned up. Air filters put in. There are home detection systems for carbon monoxide and radon. Molds can be cleaned out. Water can be filtered. Flourescent lights can be turned off and a lamp set up with bright light bulbs in them. Getting outside and breathing fresh air is beneficial. All these things can be changed. You don't have to be exposed to them.

C. MECHANICAL

We've all been bumped and bruised physically in our lives from falls, car wrecks, accidents. These seem obvious. But other mechanical trauma can occur in more subtle ways. A pillow that is not right for your neck. A bed too firm or mushy for your back. Your office chair or sitting in front of a computer all day. Lifting. Driving. Physical labor. Not enough exercise or stretching. Being overweight. These all take their toll on your bones. You more than likely have:

1. Neck pain

2. Back pain

3. Carpal Tunnel like symptoms

4. Numbness in the extremities

5. Ringing in the ears

6. Headaches/ Migraines

7. Blurry vision or vertigo

Again these things should be tended to. An ergonomic chair at work. Stretching and exercising regularly. Body therapies and chiropractic care. Taking breaks during long drives by getting out and walking a bit. Proper lifting. Losing weight.

A Note on Dental: The importance of good, routine dental care has come to light. Swollen, red, inflamed gums, plaque, tartar, tooth decay, and abcesses seriously tax the immune system constantly. Not only that, all the bacteria in the gums and teeth are right there next to a good blood supply that is feeding that bacteria straight into the body. They have linked heart disease as well as other diseases to poor dental hygiene. A good way to demonstrate how ugly the bacteria are in a human's mouth is to see the list of "infectious bite" categories. At the top of the list of severity, number 1 is human, above dog, cat, monkey or even pig. I think the only creature that tops humans for the most nasty mouth is the Komodo Dragon.

Yes, the bad news, again, is daily hygiene......brushing and flossing. Another routine. Then there are the professional cleanings by a dental hygienist at least twice a year. This will give you the best insurance for better overall health as well as keeping your teeth for a lifetime. Why is that important you may ask? Or maybe you aren't asking and just saying "hey fuck that, let them pull them all out and I'll get dentures!" Yeah, you think that's a better answer than having your own teeth?

I had a dental hygienist inform me (and inspire me through fear) that people who have dentures have a shorter life span because they tend to not be able to chew their food as well.

Chewing food well is what extracts the nutrients out of food. Now we've already covered the importance of nutrients, so I shouldn't have to explain that.

D. EMOTIONAL

What are your relationships like? Are they harmonious and joyful or are they tumultuous? Do you have close friends you can be yourself with and who understand you? Do you get along with your parents? Your spouse? Your children?

What are your finances? Are you in huge debt? Or are you getting along comfortably?

How satisfied are you with your work situation? Are you stuck? Or do you like what you are doing? Is your boss an asshole? Or are you fortunate to have a nice one at the helm?

Do you have any legal battles going on?

Are you haunted by past events in your life?

Are you suffering from any loss or grieving over losing someone dear?

These all spell STRESS. Stress is a killer. It eats away at your very core. It changes your body chemicals into acid that erodes you from the inside out. Without correcting the stressors in your life, changing the other things in your life could be fruitless. Hell, having the other things imbalanced in your life just adds more stress to the outside world of stress. More double-whammy shit.

There are myriad ways to change the stressful situations in your life. Only you can answer whether you need a career change, a relationship make-over, therapy for issues, debt consulting, meditation for calming, the list goes on and on. There are wonderful avenues to change your own internal environment from books to groups to motivational speakers. With the internet there is everything a person could ever want to know about anything. It just takes you deciding to find it.

Final Chit-Chat on Body Language

Once you begin to eliminate some offenders from any of the sources above, your body can begin to heal. Once it heals a bit you may begin to really feel a difference. Hopefully for the better. But two things to keep in mind. When a body begins the healing process, things may not go from zero to wonderful overnight. It can sometimes feel really crappy for awhile. It is more than likely detoxing. Those toxins have to find their way out and they go kicking and screaming out of the body. Hey, they've lost their meal ticket. They don't want to give up their cushy ride without a fight. So this will be your first challenge: to weather this storm. It's almost like a test. You have to pass it to get to the next level.

The next thing is that after you do get some cleansing and healing under your belt, should you reintroduce the offender back into your body, you may have a more significant reaction to it. Hey, your body likes being clean and healthy. Your body doesn't want that toxin back in there. Your body worked hard to get over it, it doesn't want to go through that again. So don't be surprised if your body lets you know its unhappiness with a much louder voice in the future.

Chapter 9: Optical Delusion

Some delusions aren't bad.....that is, it's OK to think you're Napolean Bonaparte as long as you're not hurting anyone. But what about the self deluded things we believe? Or the things we refuse to see? If we don't see it, then it doesn't exist. Isn't that kind of an optical delusion?

We all see what we want to see. Our perception is our reality. You could have the most gorgeous body, but if you truly believe you are a fat pig you will be obsessed with dieting and worse. Hence the birth of the diagnosis of anorexia nervosa. A mental condition that has actually ended with someone starving themself to death. Their perception was their reality. There is nothing more real than dead.

Yes it would be great if western medicine could look up from their microscopes and prescription pads and see the whole person. If they could look at the entire being, what goes on around him. What does he ingest, breathe, think and feel? Again, more optical delusions, this time coming from our physicians, seeing only a disease and treating the symptoms not the cause. And not the whole person.

However it may be a long time before our society gets with the program. So only you are in charge of you. It is up to you to really see, to really listen, to really feel what is inside of you. Only you can change it. If we can change ourselves then we can help others to change also. That's how this will happen. Like a ripple in the water. You are the pebble dropped into the pond. What will your ripple tell everyone else about you? Will your ripple uplift other people or drag them down into the muck?

Your brain is the most powerful drug ever. You can change yourself and change the world. Are we going to go to hell in a hand basket or are we going to find our wings and fly up to the clouds with all the other beautiful creatures in the sky? I don't care how tired my arms get, I'm going to keep flapping them because I just know there's a pair of wings back there somewhere. Even if I look like the bumbling Blue-Footed Booby, I'm still going to get airborne. (Now there's a delusion for you. But who does it hurt? Or benefit?)

CHAPTER 10: CONGRATULATIONS, YOU MADE THE SHIT LIST

The information I've been presenting in this book is not new information, nor is it difficult to acquire. This information is so prevalent now even the most cognitively impaired person has it at their fingertips. If you wish to find out more, then you will seek it out.

However, if you do not wish to do so, then let's tell our contestants what they've won, Bob.

Should you continue with the sedentary lifestyle, the eating sugary, starchy, salty, trans-fatty foods, chugging sodas and alcohol, inhaling cigarette smoke, disrespecting your sleep, filling the air with your whining, bitching and moaning, while remaining full of shit, here are the top 10 prizes you could win on our show today:

1. Obesity

2. Diabetes

3. Coronary artery disease

4. Stroke

5. Auto-immune diseases

6. Pulmonary disease

7. Osteoporosis

8. Liver disease

9. Kidney failure

10. Cancer

But don't be discouraged if you weren't one of our top winners today. There are more prizes we'll be sending home with all the participants in our showroom audience. Each one of you may be going home with:

Ulcers, IBS, constipation, acid reflux, hiatal hernias, bowel obstructions, pancreatitis, joint pain, muscles spasms, low energy, lack of motivation, mood swings, irritability, attention deficit, lack of focus, weight gain, chest pains, headaches, poor eyesight, blindness, ringing in ears, chronic infections, sinusitis, low thyroid, bad gall bladders, arthritis, bone degeneration, Alzheimer's, clogged arteries, insulin resistance, peripheral artery disease, inflammation, and the list goes on, and on.

Chapter 11: What Are You Still Doing Here?

OK, so you made it through the book. Amazing. I'd have to commend you for having some real testicles there. I might have to admit I'm impressed even. Hell, I might even think highly of you. My opinion of you could be that you are not some piece of shit melding into the couch, blaming everyone else for the miserable condition of your life. Great.

I didn't expect most cretins to get past the introduction. Hey, if you're female and got past the part on PMS, you just may be a real woman. If you are, would you do me a favor and start cloning yourself so we can begin to repopulate the earth with a stronger breed? Thanks.

So, now what are you going to do with the information? I am curious. You see, if you did get anything out of it, you may just go on to become all fabulous and shit. Then, it just might be contagious. Oh God!! A new epidemic of vibrant, thriving people!!??? Human beings getting healthy and happy? What would I do? I'd have nothing to bitch about. Nothing to write about. Hey, that would shut me up.

Alright, so where do we go from here.............

CHAPTER 12: SELF INVENTORY

I cringe at the word "change." I resist change at all costs. The fact is, that we change regardless of whether we want to or not. Even not choosing to change will still result in undergoing transformations that may not be beneficial to our well-being. Why not have a say in which direction that change may take?

I have always used lists to help me remember things and stay on track. This list would be taking an inventory of your condition. If you can see where you are at then you can map out where you are going.

Here are some general questions that will paint a picture of you now:

What is your height and weight?

What are your measurements?

What is your BMI?

What are your typical eating habits? (It is a good idea to write a daily log of *exactly* what you've ingested for several days. You might be surprised what sneaks in there.) This will require a small notepad or journal. Be very honest with yourself. This is for your own benefit not mine. If you consume alcohol, write it down.

Do you smoke?

Do you take recreational drugs?

What prescribed medications do you take?

What Over-the-Counter medications, vitamins or supplements (including herbs) do you take?

What movement do you get each week?

What is your ability to be mobile? (In other words, are you restricted by joint problems, etc.?)

What are your bowel habits? (How often do you go and what is the consistency)

Do you live with pain? Rate it on 0 - 10 each day.

What do you do to relieve that pain?

What are your menstrual cycles like (if this applies)?

Are they regular?

What is the condition of your teeth?

How is your eyesight?

How is your hearing?

Do you have any allergies?

How is your sleep?

>Do you fall asleep OK?

>Do you stay asleep?

>Do you snore or stop breathing?

Has a Doctor diagnosed you with any conditions?

Were any tests or labwork done?

Do you understand what the results of those tests meant?

Do you have any family history of diseases or mental illness?

Have you ever had a head injury?

Do you see a Dentist regularly?

What is the condition of your teeth?

What are your Stressors?

> Finances?
>
> Job?
>
> Relationships?
>
> Diet?
>
> Health Issues?

Any other issues that create stress (these can even be good things like planning a wedding or going to school)

What is your basic mood?

> Does it change?
>
> How?
>
> When? (daily, weekly, monthly?)
>
> Do you know why it changes?

How do you deal with your emotions?

Where do you live?

> What kind of lifestyle is that? (ie. crowded polluted city, open rural area, etc.)

Who do you live with?

Do you have a sexual outlet?

    Is it safe?

What do you do for fun?

Do you have Spiritual support?

What are your hobbies?

So you get the idea. Anything you can ask yourself that gives you a "snapshot" of who you are right now. It's easy to look at other people and see what's wrong with them or even what's right. It's not so easy to do it with ourselves. It takes courage and brutal honesty. We run from it. It's funny because usually our bad habits, like overeating or drinking, are what we do to numb the feelings of having to look at ourselves. But, you have to look at yourself in order to rectify those bad habits, and what they've done to you that have caused the problems of why you are having to look at yourself. If you know there is something that is not right, here's where you have to be totally naked in front of the mirror, literally and figuratively. It's only going to get worse if you don't face it now.

Chapter 13: Transformation
OR
"The C Word"

No, not that word. I just didn't want to use the word change again. It has a bad taste the way the word diet does. It means suffering, loss, deprivation. But a caterpillar doesn't mind transforming into a butterfly, does he or she? If you can add a little something into your fixed way of perceiving the world, each day, then you can expand and transform. It can actually be quite painless. Hell, you'll probably even BE pain free and feeling downright good. Shit, what a concept!

This is where you ask yourself, "how motivated am I?" Can you commit to new ways? (Uh-Oh, another "C" word). Do you grasp that it is a life commitment and not some 2 week starvation boot camp and then it will all be over? Do you really get what it means if you don't alter some of those destructive ways? Do you need the reality of a board upside your head before you get the "ah ha" you need to change? Like having to stick a needle in your massively obese thigh everyday with medication that will eventually lead to the infamous "them" cutting off parts of your body from broken down blood vessels, cellulitis and gangrene? Add to that, kidney failure or going blind. Keep eating that non-nutritive, processed food, drinking a river of soda, sitting on that ass with its own zip code, and you'll be well on your way to saying hello to that two by four headed for your noggin.

Alright, so you've made it this far. Lets look at the most important thing. Solutions. What would some of those shifts look like? What could be a first step? Look back at some of the questions. You could put it into categories.

A. EATING. Check your answers. Were there a lot of the things I had spelled out as non-nutritive food stuffs? Remember, this is not going to be a diet. This will be a life sustaining maintenance plan. There will be no deprivation. These new food choices will all switch to "what I can have" and "all that I want" types of food. Once your body receives nutritive foods it will stop craving the non-nutritive crap that makes you voracious in search for nutrients and just keeps packing on the pounds while at the same time craving even more crap.

B. EXERCISE. Yes, I know, another four letter word. Some form of moving your body. Some form of resistance. Cardio and muscle toning of some kind. Even if you are in a wheelchair, you can do aerobics with just arm movements. You can tone muscles without the use of weights with isometrics. If you sit in a chair all day at work, clench your muscles, shrug your shoulders, roll your eyes. If you can take breaks and go for a walk, that's even better. There are many 5 to 10 minute workouts all over YouTube. Starting your day with a brisk short workout will change everything from your brain on down to your toes. Without motion and strength, everything will deteriorate.

C. SLEEP. If you aren't getting this, your brain and everything else will suffer. It could be as easy as just forming new habits like turning off the TV or it can be as complex as figuring out if you are in some adrenal-stress-blood sugar-melatonin chess game and you are losing. The bottom line is you have to get some sleep no matter where and when, for however long you can get it. You're fighting a two-headed monster here. Your internal reasons why you can't sleep and society's whip to be driven and not honor one of life's greatest necessities. Block out the second one. Society doesn't give two shits about whether you live or die. And die miserably. So screw them and stand up (or lie down, I should say) for what you need.

D. DENTAL. This is self explanatory. Much of our health is affected by our dental condition. So it needs to be tended to.

E. MENTAL. Your thoughts, your emotions, your stress levels. These all affect our hormones. And usually not good hormones either. Adrenal stress is at the basis of many destructive processes in our bodies. If it is not kept in check this is another slippery slope. How can you build in mini vacations for your mind? Where can you find sanctuary from the barrage of thoughts and images that come at us all day like a crazed batting cage ball launcher that's gone haywire? Yes, drinking is fun and is good for an occasional treat, but it is not a good long term friend.

F. PURPOSE. What is your purpose in life? Do you know? If you feel you have a purpose, it will motivate you in so many aspects of your life. You'll want to stay healthy so you can fulfill your destiny. You are here for a reason. Don't waste it. If you haven't figured it out, then I urge you to be giving it some thought. In this day and age of self help there are many people out there who can help you in self discovery. Even God himself could, if you ask.

Consider this......you could be "stuffing" or avoiding with some other non-productive activity (like over-spending or even PTA Queen) because deep down it is too scary or too much work (or both) to ferret out who you are. Sometimes that "true self" lies behind a wall of demons. We all have them. Big and small. Just remember, if you choose not to deal with them, they will be steering your ship. You can only release their death grip on that wheel if you illuminate them with focus and acceptance. They hate the light. Once you shine that spotlight on them then you can shine.

Here's another concept. Demons, toxins and fat all congregate together. Chasing out the demons (issues), ceasing to put toxins in your mouth (saying no to processed foods) and exercise will allow fat to breakdown and be released. Remember that fat harbors toxins? Fat is also a psychological buffer when we are wounded. So this could be why finding your purpose could be scary. You'd be dealing with issues while taking responsibility for yourself and your health. Wow, that just sounds like too much work. I'm too busy making a living and taking care of my family, you might say. We all are. But a man who says he'll try finds excuses and a man who says he will finds a way.

What Could Be Your First Step?

Buy a journal you like and start a food diary.

Try watching some documentaries on real food choices.

Buy some fresh vegetables at the health food store or farmer's market.

Try drinking one large glass of fresh water for every soda you drink.

Try eating some nuts instead of a candy bar. (As long as you are not allergic).

Try eating eggs in the morning instead of cereal or a bagel. (Or a piece of chicken or tuna).

Try some jumping jacks for 5 minutes in the morning or on a break.

Try to go to bed before 10 PM with the TV off.

Keep a journal by the bed to write down any nagging thoughts.

Investigate vitamin supplements.

Floss your teeth each day.

Buy a used treadmill, stationary bike or trampoline.

Try some gluten free bread or pasta.

Purchase some grass fed beef.

Talk to a counselor or minister if you have troubling feelings.

Accept yourself just as you are right now.

Research the power of forgiveness.

Write down one small thing you can do today. (It's up to you to do it).

I bid you farewell and God's grace. Let all you do for yourself trickle down to the next generation and the earth, that we will continue to be welcome upon this beautiful planet that has been more than gracious about our assault upon her.

Some Reference Suggestions

Documentaries:

Hungry for Change

Fat, Sick and Nearly Dead

Food Matters

Super Size Me

Books:

Eat Right 4 Your Type by Dr. D'Adamo

Is Your Child's Brain Starving by Dr. Michael Lyons

Fit or Fat by Covert Bailey

5 Day Miracle Diet by Adele Puhn

Websites:

PubMed.gov

    (for over 107, 000 articles on Oxidative Stress)

TheABCvideo.com or on YouTube

    (the answer to oxidative stress)

MyLifeVantage.com/patriciaadonahue

    (where to purchase Protandim)

KeepItMovingFitness.com

Herbal Healer Academy.com

    (for good quality products)

Movies: (Funny but no joke)

Wall.e

Idiocracy

www.ingramcontent.com/pod-product-compliance
Lightning Source LLC
Chambersburg PA
CBHW021624270326
41931CB00008B/852